AF472372

ENOUGH IS ENOUGH
FINALLY

A REAL WAY TO GET PERMANENT WEIGHT LOSS

CHRISTOPHER L. EADDY, PHD, NLP

Cover: Justice Dan Jake
Editing Support: Ceri Usmar
Contributors: Clair, PhD, Joseph McClendon, Deepak Chopra, (Anthony "Dietzy" Bertone, Daniel Pritchard, Kevin Candido – The Circle, Dr. K. Fredlund)

ISBN: 978-1-5136-1383-3 (sc)
ISBN: 978-1-5136-1385-7 (e)

Eyes Wide Open Publishing
Raleigh NC 27610
855-600-9090
Third Eye Publishing

Lulu Publishing Services rev. date: 04/02/2019

Disclaimer

This book is designed to get you to think differently, not just generally, but at a subconscious level. It is written with generous uses of improper tense to allow your brain to open recall files and make associations to the past and future thoughts almost without you noticing. It is designed to create sensations, unconscious connections, and thought provoking images that you can follow along with mentally. Be careful to read for content so as not to miss the forest for the trees. This book seeks to get you results which cannot come with traditional means or you would have already had them.

It is not meant to be a replacement for professional medical advice or counseling although much of the information has been observed and influenced by both. Of course, if you have questions about what you read, ask your primary provider for their opinion.

For Irene, Dennis, Kevin, Valerie, Lee, Alexis, Collin, Jeanie, Horacio, Aaron, Danny, Ralph, Maurice, Brent Campbell, Ivalesse, Lynne, Elvin, Vinny, Dr. K. Fredlund, K. Pernell, Troy, Dr. Brad Butler, Dee Best, Dr. Candice Carlisle-Roberts, Dr. Brian Nunez, Sherrie, Sandra, Joseph, Jennifer, Roy Lee, Elvin, Dennis, Moses, Edna, Ricky and Steve, George, Ruby, PJ, Derrick, Consuela, Roger, Red, Omar, and Cheesburger

(Motivation, Information, Encouragement, Patience, Listening, Feedback, Time, Dialogue)

Contents

Author's Note

I am constantly learning more about the subject of human healthiness and how to live without being overweight or obese. In return, I passionately and persuasively share what I learn, especially when I can validate its reliability and truthfulness through experience and overwhelming data.

The idea that health and weight and even the idea that weight-loss, however it is defined, is critical to our world's health, and self-preservation should not be surprising. How we view the ideas of our health, especially if we are overweight, fat or obese, influences our job status, our health costs, and our social and emotional well-being.

So, it is the gist of this writing, and my hope, that you will gain your motivation towards great results that lead you to better manage your weight, a healthier perspective on your weight, your food intake, and your overall health in general while reading this book. Most importantly I know it will give you clarity about weight loss itself.

It will be critical for understanding that as you read this book, you will come across several strange writing conventions. They are purposeful and have intended meaning.

I am excited and grateful to all of those who have been willing to answer my pestering questions and my forward – almost annoying – style and approach to wondering why people around me do what they do, eat what they eat, say what they say, and believe what they believe. It has helped me and allowed me to study how to share what I have learned, and think through what I believe. It has been an incredible journey to complete this book. Know that I am grateful to those of you who allowed me to "confront" you and pick your brain to fortify my own thinking. Thank you.

May this writing and the seminars that support it enhance and improve your well-being and your healthiness like never before and beyond your expectations.

Christopher

Foreword

When this transcript was first written, I was double majoring in a Nursing and a Health/Fitness degree, long after my earlier degrees. I shared the book with some of my classmates. One of them was thoroughly offended saying I had presumed to know what was inside her head and did not like my approach.

Although that was not the case and is impossible at best, it made me wonder about how I was writing this book. After studying the issues around weight reduction, understanding my own concerns about my own healthiness; I had to be sure I was genuine and empathetic with those with whom this book would be shared. I decided to experiment and gain some weight, believing I could easily take the weight off at will, and at the least, be more compassionate about what I was writing.

My primary care doctor was my neighbor, and after several visits with him and some lengthy conversations, I set out to experience life beyond being fit. I say fit because I had played football in high school (Bishop Maginn, Albany NY) and played college football (at Temple University – Go Owls!). So, I knew how to build muscle, exercise, and eat somewhat healthy to be fit.

The experiment was a different animal, though. My weight started to rise from 228 and over an extended period (7 months to a year), I had placed almost 100 pounds onto my frame. In some of those conversations with my Doctor, he was highly concerned about my blood pressure which was now moving through the acceptable range into the borderline range and he expressed concern about whether I was making a good decision. At 324 pounds I knew it had gone long enough and it was time to change course.

Unable to wear clothes off of the rack at local clothing stores, aching joints, lacking flexibility, binge eating, processed foods, eating around the clock, a lack of motivation to exercise regularly, and even wearing bigger clothes to hide the overages, I was growing weary. I was easily tired, had heart palpitations, night sweats, incredible pain in my knees and even headaches that required neurologist and physical therapy visits. At the pinnacle of my weight gain experiment with no clear end in sight, and no clear path for how I was going to reverse course, I read an article in a Readers Digest. In the article, the former very overweight athlete-writer spoke about eating uncontrollably (whole pizzas, bottles of wine, cake and sweets, hot dogs, pastas, and even steaks,) all in the same day. He spoke about how tough it was to really reduce his size after allowing himself to get to the weight at which he was to play his sport. ("Boy, could I relate for different reasons…"). Then he shared what we all must do if we want the results of being our best, being healthier, and fit too; just do it, grit through it and be ok doing whatever it takes to be healthier.

After reading that article over and over for several days, I started my quest for healthiness and not just fitness. I began walking and researching the topic even more. I began to see small differences, but it wasn't enough. After working in the local emergency department and having a few upsetting experiences, I was through with the extra weight forever. As a result of what I saw and learned, I was able to drop almost 100 pounds fairly rapidly and have helped countless others to see that dropping the fat has to occur in a precise way in the thought process *first.* I do not presume to know what is in your head. However, if you are like me and want to live life fully, as soon as possible, then you'll agree that what you read here may be the easiest and most permanent way to get those results.

Chapter One

Two-and-a-Half Magic Thoughts

Because Nobody Gets Out Alive

News Flash!

You're going to die! That is a reality for all of us. Barring any accident or disaster, the slowest way to meet this fate is to be as healthy as possible… (and why wouldn't you?)

In today's world, most of us are aware of some of the information that exists, regarding what it means to be healthy. Unfortunately, most of us know what to do, because we tend to read and listen to the messages we get daily, but rarely do we do all that we know, we are supposed to do.

So, where is the-disconnect; what is the problem?

What is the reason our waistlines keep expanding? Why are there so many of us who have and are going through the "bigger me" phase in life?

Perhaps, one of the major issues with being healthy is how we think about healthiness itself. In spite of the many views that exist about it, the main consideration that determines our healthiness is how we treat our bodies. In many cases, the issues of healthiness begin with what we eat and our levels of exercise. This is what helps us regulate our weight and our best efforts in getting slender when we've allowed ourselves to become overweight and fat.

The good news is that this is something we can overcome, regardless of how big we are or have allowed ourselves to become. It's not as difficult as it seems and can be *really* easy to achieve. I mean really easy if you are willing to be informed and then commit to act on what you learn. I promise, that if you have tried in the past without results, what you will learn as you read this book is that you were just not going after it correctly!

To Get Great Results- you must Get Started

~CLE

There are *only two-and-a-half simple things* you don't have in your mind, or you'd be fit and healthy right now; you'd be your ideal weight (or the weight you choose to be), and you would have no concerns about your weight in the future.

As soon as you put these two and a half thoughts in your mind, you'll start getting slender without even thinking about it. Of course, you can expedite your results to be healthier, fit and less overweight with some additional effort, but you won't have to be concerned about it anymore. You won't feel deprived when you don't eat certain things and in fact you'll feel like you're eating like a king or queen! You'll feel like you're stuffing yourself! And you'll be able to stop eating long before you experience that "I'm really full feeling."

These two-and-a-half simple thoughts are mostly what we'd call neuro-*imagination* thoughts (thoughts that create neurological patterns). And you'll enjoy the heck out of seeing yourself in this new way full of possibilities to be healthy for the rest of your life. You'll get to see what is, the way you thought it never was. By the way, it won't be any big overwhelming change; and, "Guess what," Because it is simple and not a big change, your mind will "sop" these thoughts right up like a big thirsty sponge! As I mentioned, it's somewhat easy with the correct thoughts in your head.

I'm going to show you how to get these two-and-a-half magic thoughts into your mind in a way a 10-year-old would. I'll show you how to easily keep them there. Then, without even thinking about your weight, you'll begin to gradually become the healthier you – all while concentrating on enjoying your visit to this wonderful world we live in.

As you probably know already, there's a lot of people who want you to rearrange a large part of your life to be healthier; some want you to take so-called weight loss supplements, or undergo rigorous exercise routines that are often painful and sometimes unhealthy. Others may recommend things like surgery, which has its place in the grand scheme of healthiness. Often, however, surgery does not yield the results it is supposed to and is typically deemed successful if the person only gains back less than 50% or less of the weight the surgery helped take off.

The circumstance you're in and the emotions you feel as a result, is not the end of your journey. The evidence is there, that things change and no matter what you think, you can experience better and have the best of what can be.

~CLE

To be the healthiest you – You have to be free from issues related to your weight and what comes along with being overweight. This can happen when you have, the two-and-a-half simple thoughts in your mind to get you moving in the most precise direction. This is all but your guarantee to make sure your efforts and results get achieved.

I've done a lot of studying on the topic. I've got several degrees, licenses, certifications, a Ph.D. and several other letters behind my name. In spite of that, all of this studying has done little for me regarding becoming healthier. What I have discovered as a result however, is that behind anything we really want to do, is a simple core change we have to make. It is never anything big or complicated; never anything that would take a Ph.D. to figure out. It's simple, and rather easy once we understand the process of how to do it.

That's right; I said easy. See, the reason I say easy and only two-and-a-half thoughts, is because you already have half of the third thought in your mind. All you have to do is complete it. So, you only need to have two completely new thoughts and the completion of the third and you're on the way to being a smaller you.

Now if you're wondering why this is any different from anything you have tried and why you're previous efforts didn't work as you had hoped, it's this: "Without these two complete thoughts and the completion of the third, nothing is going to work."

Once you have these two-and-a-half thoughts in your mind, you will begin to notice small yet important changes occurring. You'll wake up now, on the first morning after reading this book wondering what the new feeling you are having is all about. It will intrigue you such that **you** will have wanted to read Enough is Enough twice, to make sure you have missed nothing (when you **do read it now!**)

If you tried to achieve significant weight loss before and it didn't work out for you then, this is what you've been waiting for. This is the way to get real results without all of the hype and false promises. And for some of you – the change is already being felt, now. It begins in your thoughts with hopefulness and anticipation that you have found the answer.

Sometimes thinking out of the box is not enough. We have to be ok doing non-traditional things that get us the results we want.

~CLE

Your thoughts are critical because they prompt your beliefs. Your beliefs are your foundation that prompts your desires (your want to's). These desires prompt your actions by which you judge yourself. Your actions become the content of your character. Ultimately, your character defines who You Are – Changing.

In preparation for having the TWO-AND-A-HALF MAGIC THOUGHTS embedded into your mind, we need to look at some general considerations that act as preparation or a platform for the thoughts to reside on and in. First and foremost is how to read this book and get the most out of it.

So depending on how you normally read, this may be helpful and or at the least guiding, in terms of a way you might want to read this book . . . First, do not read this book as a 1. Study guide, 2. a Devotional, 3. as an Editor or 4. as a Stretch read. (1. STUDY GUIDE –With the intent of being memorized for later recall to prove competency 2. DEVOTIONAL a daily meditation or spiritual practice guide 3. EDITOR- grammar, punctuation, proofing, single sentence/paragraph read and applying the backwards test, 4. STRETCH reading for the knowledge of who has written it and their bibliography as well as their sources)

Instead, consider this perspective. Read this book with the intention of getting new results for yourself. Read this book with the anticipation that it will provide information that will motivate you and excite you to be your best, healthiest you. Read this book with a willingness to try on what is asked of you as if it were new, well-fitted clothing that you wanted. Then, if it does not work for you, negate it. Also, play full out in the exercises you're asked to do – do them and you will gain so much more value and the unconscious work that this book is designed to give you will have its best chance at giving you the results you want.

Ignore the stuff that seems to be written in a weird way. Some of it is subconscious commands, sparks to the imagination and even completion of previous chapter's thoughts or the opening for ones that will be completed later. Remember to get something you don't have and perhaps have never had you have to do something different and maybe something you might not have ever had to do.

Read; Explore; Respond; Apply; Repeat if necessary –

Secondly, there are quotes smattered throughout the book. The way I recommend using them is with each chapter find one that resonates with you or find one that you feel has some meaning and value and write it down or creatively duplicate it so you can see it often for a week at a minimum. Use them as motivational cues, repeat them mentally, verbally or even adopt them as a philosophy. (Ultimately, you are rewriting your brain's "hard drive")

Lastly, this book will build from a foundation of information, some of which you may already know to a heavier dose of do's, don'ts and considerations. Try to avoid negating the basics even if it is review. If the information is not new to you and you are not implementing it as an active part of your life, when is now a good time to start using it?

Chapter Two

Should You Consider Taking off the Extra Weight

Becoming healthy is not just some theory based, ideal way of thinking or being.

It's not something that was thought up by health fanatics, medical personnel, Hollywood, the food industry, or even the weight loss industry itself. It's not a way of shaping our bodies, so we look a certain way to impress others or even the act of starving ourselves to "lose weight."

It's about living longer and enjoying the life we have, without disease and limitation due to health problems caused by being overweight or fat. To get to this almost mysterious state of healthiness and especially, if we are overweight or fat requires us to be honest and take a close look at a few facts and some things that we need to know more about. Some of these considerations should help us decide or at least seriously consider why we should focus our attention on the issue of taking off the extra weight in the first place.

Here are some of those considerations (some facts of reality) that we have to take into account.

We need fat in our bodies to survive. Once we have too much fat to benefit our body's functions and its purposes-we are not only hurting our health and our body, but we begin the process of slowly killing ourselves.

The effects of too much fat are simple. More fat means more body mass (bigger body). The bigger your body, the more blood is required to keep it alive. The more blood you need, *the harder your heart has to work* to move "more blood" around. Unlike exercise which strengthens the heart muscle, this harder working heart is not strengthening, it is being stressed or is straining to keep up with pushing the blood, nutrients and oxygen around in your circulatory system. Also the excess fat stored in our bodies, especially in our waists tends to attach to our vital organs in and around our torso (between our shoulders and groin). This causes our organs to strain in their ability to function and makes them less efficient, and eventually they fail to work.

I know it sounds a bit brutal and direct, however, it is just the fact of reality that we have to face when it comes to being overweight. We are killing ourselves, and this is the main consideration.

Other considerations:

Fact #1: Every pound of fat is equal to approximately 3500 calories

This means, if you want to begin the process of "burning fat off your body," then we have to create a negative in your food intake. Here's another way to look at it. Your body has calories in it and every day we add even more calories to it. What we have to do is force the body to use more of the calories we've already stored rather than what we consume daily.

For Example:

You eat 2500 calories daily	2500
You walk for an hour and burn 500	-500
You only need 1500 calories	-1000
You store an excess of 500 calories in your body	+1000

These extra calories get stored in the body and are stored as fat. So not regulating your caloric intake is the perfect recipe for creating fat and being over fat and even obese with time.

To begin the reduction of fat in the human body, you have to know or have some approximate idea of how many calories based on your BMI (Body Mass Index) you should be consuming. Knowing how much you need to consume to be healthy helps you determine how much you can safely reduce your eating portions so that your 500 calories burned begins to use up the actual stored calories in your body, so, it would work in the instance, where you could consume on any given "normal" day 2000 calories instead.

What's even better is if you could consume 1500 to 1700 calories on a low activity day and burn your normal 500 calories walking, you would be creating a caloric deficit or "negative storage" and your body would have to burn calories that are stored in the body.

This is the beginning of the change that is often called "weight loss." This is where the weight begins to come off and obviously, the greater the deficit, the faster the weight reduction; so, you could engage in more rigorous exercise, burning more calories, creating a greater deficit. And as we know and agreed upon already, we're not "losing it" we're getting rid of it-permanently.

Fact #2

There is no specific food that is going to make you burn calories faster than some other food. Although there is information that says some foods can increase your metabolic rate; making you burn more calories, this is not completely true. This "hype" type of information has been out in the real world for quite some time with absolutely no significant results that all can agree on. While different foods offer different health benefits, people are often left wondering if calories burned, vary from one food to the next.

Ultimately, "A calorie is a calorie, regardless of where it comes from," says Elizabeth Pivonka, Ph.D., RD, President of the Produce for Better Health Foundation. There are no foods that increase your metabolic rate, or help you burn calories, she says. Even if certain foods do increase your metabolism, the amount is too insignificant to make it a magic bullet or something you can rely on consistently. She recommends that you eat foods with a high water and fiber content because they stay in your system longer, and you won't want to eat as often which is a plus for taking off the pounds. (Real information from a Registered Dietician, not the magazine or television/internet hype designed to sell you something).

Having said that, and having experienced all of what she's said-both trying different foods to boost metabolism and eating more fiber balanced meals, I will admit that there have been some hot pepper moments when my body was certainly operating at a hotter temperature while I was sitting still, (dripping sweat), and my metabolism was in fact prompted to try and regulate my body to a cooler state. That is a momentary and interpreted state of increased metabolic activity yet is not a sustainable state of metabolism increase to be able to tout it as food that consistently increases metabolism for two reasons.

The whole world steps aside for the person who knows where he or she is going.[1]

~ James Allen

One – the body is amazing in its ability to build up a tolerance to things we ingest and to the weight we gain. So, to get long-term metabolic increases you'd have to increase your pepper (Capsaicin) intake constantly and secondly, because peppers create peristalsis (poop onset) you would have to be so careful to eat in a way that helps you retain the nutrients from the food you eat before it quickly leaves your body as waste.

Fact #3

Excess weight is the leading underlying cause of Type II diabetes. However, there is a silver lining to this sobering news: weight reduction not only can help prevent the onset of diabetes but may also improve the health of people who already have the disorder.

Fact #4

There is a serious cost (literally and figuratively) to being over fat or obese. Let's examine a few of them closely so we are diligently informed in making our decisions to be healthier people.

How much obesity must we create in a single decade for us to realize that it ain't just diet, but our mentality, language and lack of desire to change it, that is the cause?

~CLE

Cost #1 – Your Risk of cancer:

Dr. Raul Seballos, Vice Chairman of Preventive Medicine at the Cleveland Clinic and an affiliate of The National Cancer Institute Associates, notes that there are 34,000 new cases of cancer in men and 50,000 in women who have obesity each year.

He states, "It could be that excess fat cells increase hormonal activity or they increase growth factors that lead to tumor growth. Obese people are at higher risk for all cancers," Seballos said. "They are often diagnosed in later stages of cancer than thinner people and are more likely to die from the disease."

Cost #2 – The Risk to the unborn child:

A new study in the Journal of the American Medical Association found that obesity increases a woman's chance of having a preterm baby, especially when her body mass index is 35 or higher. The study's authors speculate that having too much fat may inflame and weaken the uterine and cervical membranes. Whatever the reason, it can have devastating effects. Premature birth is the leading cause of infant death and long-term disabilities.

Cost #3 – Less Sleep and Lower Quality of Sleep

If you are overweight or obese, your sleep and your weight are not going to be a good partnership if you are not getting enough of it. Nearly 80 percent of older, obese Americans report having problems with sleep, a recent American Sleep Foundation survey found.

Poor sleep contributes to a host of diseases including diabetes, heart disease and, ironically, *obesity itself.* Numerous studies link shortened sleep and less quality sleep to expanding waistlines, including the Harvard Nurses' Study, which found that those who slept less than five hours a night were 15 percent more likely to gain weight than those who enjoyed at least seven hours of sleep.

Dr. Donald Hensrud, a nutritionist and preventive medicine expert in the department of endocrinology, diabetes, metabolism and nutrition at the Mayo Clinic said, "One of the most immediate health dangers for many obese people is sleep apnea, a condition in which a person gasps or stops breathing momentarily while asleep."

As I have learned from Dr. K Fredlund, MD, (KF) to the contrary of poor sleep, that great sleep involves, proper mindset, correct sleep environment and even lighting considerations when we awake in the middle of the night to use the bathroom, etc.

Being overweight and obese are major risk factors for many chronic diseases for all Americans. When people are overweight or obese, they have more health problems in general and more serious health problems as well. Additionally, there are higher healthcare costs.

~CLE

"Sleep apnea can be caused by increased fat around the neck area that presses down and closes off the soft tissues of the airways while a person is lying down, especially on his back," Hensrud said. "This means the person does not get good quality sleep, has less oxygen in the blood stream, and the heart has to work harder" (not to mention the effects on the low amount of oxygen to the brain).

Cost #4 – Financial Costs:

A George Washington University School of Public Health study found a strong connection between greater obesity and shrinking wages. Examining data from the 2004 National Longitudinal Survey of Youth, researchers discovered that wages among the obese were $8,666 less for females and $4,772 lower for males compared with their thinner counterparts. In 2008, the researchers found wages were $5,826 less for obese females – a 14.6 percent penalty over normal-weight females.

Slimmer females, especially, do seem to have fatter wallets. In a University of Florida study, women who weighed 25 pounds less than the group average, earned $15,572 a year more than women of normal weight and women who tipped the scales at 25 pounds above the average weight earned an average of $13,847 less than an average weight female.

One should eat to live,
not live to eat.[2]
~Moliere

MAJOR CONSIDERATION #2

IS OUR FOOD MAKING YOU FAT?

I had the honor of reading, listening to and meeting Dr. William Davis, MD, author of "Wheat Belly." In his writing, he asserts that there are certain foods that are causing the American population specifically to become fat.

I decided to change my eating habits as a result of the information and conduct an easy test on two occasions to validate the information. My effort was to ascertain whether I could disregard it or use it.

The major assertion in his book is that *wheat* made in the particular manner in which it is currently modified in such a way that our bodies do not handle the kinds of carbohydrates found in this modified version. Of course, we all know that certain fats and carbohydrates contribute to our body – fat concentration. In the same manner, he says that the way in which wheat is now made represents a carbohydrate structure that the body cannot easily digest and as mentioned before (the body either assimilates or eliminates anything we put into it); these carbohydrates are converted to fat and stored in the body.

With a different number of tests and studies already done and with much more needed, the initial data is somewhat convincing-perhaps this means, wheat in some forms should be a limited part of our diet.

Additionally, new data suggests that eating genetically modified corn as well as this kind of wheat can contribute to obesity as reported in women's health, February 2013. Scientists at the Norwegian veterinary college released a 10-year study demonstrating that animals fed genetically engineered or genetically modified corn got fatter quicker and retained the weight compared to animals fed a non-genetically engineered diet. The studies were performed on rats, mice, snakes and salmon, achieving the same result with each. This study has been duplicated in the US, Australia, Turkey, Ireland, Hungary, and Austria.

Your body is an input-output system. It will always give you output based on what you input. Choose carefully and purposely, what you input.

~CLE

In simple, because the digestive system detects components of the genetically engineered products and then has to work harder to digest them; the body may try to compensate for the increased work by boosting food intake.

You have to take the time in life to know that what you are being told or sold is actually good for you, rather than being persuaded by popular opinion or great marketing messages.

~ CLE

Chapter Three

Getting Around the Weight Loss Challenge

To deal with the issue of fat, as it relates to being overweight or obese, there are several things that you have to know and understand to be able to make significant, lasting changes in your health. The information in this chapter alone should give you a good foundation for understanding some things that are beneficial for you and some things that are detrimental to you.

If you decide to use these bits of information, know that unfortunately, as I have and will continue to mention, there is no panacea, no silver bullet, no effortless (except fasting to the point of near starvation) way in which to reduce your weight. You will struggle to reduce your weight effectively – which means long-term results, unless you have a good understanding of how to manage the fat, your movement, and how to slowly taper your caloric intake.

Of course, once we've built a good base of helpful information to assist you in making your mind up about (whether you want to complete this journey of) permanent weight reduction, I will walk you through the Two and A Half Magic Thoughts that give you the results of a healthier life.

To get this lifestyle, I will offer information in this chapter that will provide you with options as you put together your strategy for how you will approach your weight reduction process. Be mindful though, Data and Research is subject to interpretation, can be made to demonstrate the author's points, and ultimately anybody's information is rarely effective for every person who reads it, does it, or is part of the studies that a lot of the data comes from.

So, if you attempt to use any of the strategies and find that any particular one does not work for you, there is no reason to be stressed about it; let it go and try another one until you find the regimen that works for you.

Let's start with a simple strategy like eating *APPLES*. In a 2003 clinical study of nearly 500 women at the State University of Rio de Janeiro, in Brazil, a 12 week study was conducted. It involved three test groups, all eating one specific food item and generally changing nothing else in their life. The study showed that women who ate three apples daily compared to those who ate pears or oat cookies, three times daily, showed a reduction in their weight, having changed no other habits after 12 weeks.

GLUTEN FREE CRAZE

Wheat-free products may be hot items in the marketplace, but that doesn't necessarily mean they are better for you, says Registered Dietitian Nutritionist Karen Ansel M.S., (coauthor of *The Calendar Diet: A Month by Month Guide to Losing Weight While Living Your Life*). Since gluten adds texture and taste to many foods, manufacturers often have to replace it with sugar, fat, and starch, which can pack more calories than the original gluten version would. "If you want to limit your intake, you are better off choosing naturally gluten-free whole foods like buckwheat, veggies, and sweet potatoes," says nutrition therapist and Registered Dietitian Limor Baum from www.nutritionenergy.com.

Every major success in healthiness comes from a collection of moments – when small decisions in each moment changes the next one – value each moment you have as an opportunity to be healthy.

~ CLE

The proof is in the ingredients, read 'em

~CLE

WRAPS

If you are looking to cut carbs, these flat seemingly wonderful bandits, appear to be a perfect solution as an alternative for sandwiches – but hold on a moment. The truth is that most of these types of alternatives have more than 275 calories before putting the fillings in it. At that calorie rate, you will have eaten almost three slices of enriched flour bread with fewer calories. Another concern is that they are typically bigger than most bread products. As a result, most wrap makers put more stuff in it than would fit in a regular sandwich. New York, Registered Dietitian Amy Shapiro, of, www.realnutritionnyc.com also points out that, "It is easy to remove the top slice of bread and eat a sandwich open-faced, but who rips off part of a wrap?" "Even wraps that are supposed to be made of spinach, tomato, and whole-wheat hardly ever have significant amounts of those things in them. Though they do contain fat," she says.

<u>SNACK MIXES</u> (granola, nuts, & other finger snacks)

At one time nuts, fruit pieces, grains and a few pieces of candy was thought to be a healthy snack (the car ride, in between classes, snack breaks in the office, etc.) Most trail mixes and granola mixes are currently made with a list of dietary woes that might make you want to consider avoiding them, things like: trans-fats, sugars, partially hydrogenated oils and even teeth damaging gooey products.

Additionally, "the nutrition information of serving size is usually a quarter of a cup of granola", says registered dietitian Laura Cipullo from lauracipullollc.com. "Most people eat up to three times that in one sitting," she explains. "But since a lot of trail mixes and granolas are made with high-calorie ingredients like maple syrup, honey, nuts, and dried fruits, that can add up to hundreds of calories." "Use a small handful as a guide to make sure you don't overdo it," she says.

<u>BRAN MUFFINS</u>

Though bran is a high-fiber and nutrient-rich carbohydrate, the amount in most bran muffins – is a mere 10 percent, according to Shapiro—

"Doesn't make up for its overall cake-like ingredient list of white flour, oil, butter, eggs, milk, and sugar. (we already know where this is going . . .) Some of these muffins don't even contain the bran or pumpernickel they advertise." Unfortunately, they use food coloring instead. "Muffins, bran or not, have anywhere from 300 to 500 calories each, so you are better off just choosing the kind you like rather than opting for a 'healthier' option that won't satisfy you," says Cipullo.

"If you want something a bit closer to the whole grain type of meal or snack there are sprout grain English muffins, which have about 160 calories and 6 grams of fat, plus 8 grams of filling protein," suggests Ansel.

Often the toughest thing to do in life is change...

-CLE

CAESAR SALAD

While getting a salad is usually a virtuous move, Caesars tend to do more harm than good. "An entrée-size salad with shaved cheese and Caesar dressing (ingredients include: cheese, eggs, oil, and salty anchovies) contains almost half of your daily fat needs and makes up a third of your daily calorie intake," says Baum. And most are made with romaine, one of the least nutritious greens there is. If a Caesar salad seems like the best menu option available, or if you're seriously craving one, ask for the dressing on the side, drizzle with just two tablespoons, and add grilled chicken or shrimp so you can balance out your meal.

FAT-FREE SALAD DRESSINGS

"When asked about fat-free dressings, I always tell my clients that it is better to use the real thing, just less of it," says Shapiro, who suggests aiming for about 1 to 2 tablespoons. "Research shows that when you eat fat-free foods, you also eat bigger portions. And when removing fat, manufacturers add extra sugar to preserve the taste." "Furthermore, your body needs fat to absorb many fat-soluble nutrients in a salad, such as lycopene from tomatoes, beta-carotene from carrots, and vitamin K in leafy greens," explains Ansel. The full-fat dressing will help you feel fuller for longer, as well as maximize the nutrition from your salad bowl.

VEGGIE CHIPS

Don't fall for their colorful and vegetable-like appearance – veggie chips aren't much better for you than regular old potato chips. That's because "most are coated in oil and salt and stripped of the majority of their nutritional value throughout the cooking process," says Baum. "One serving of veggie chips is almost nutritionally equivalent to potato chips – you get the same amount of calories and sodium with maybe only 1 or 2 fewer grams of fat," says Shapiro.

The moral of the story is: If you want veggies, eat the real thing, and if it's chips you're after, just have a small serving of them.

ENERGY BARS

These may seem like the answer to that dreaded 4 p.m. hunger induced weariness, but it's worth your while to be selective. "Energy bars provide energy through calories just like any other food," says Cipullo.

"They don't necessarily give you a different or better energy boost than a balanced meal would." But since you likely eat them because they're convenient when on-the-go, you must check the ingredients list and avoid bars with a double serving size in a single bar or lots of added sugars or fiber. Cipullo suggests Kind bars, Lara bars, Rise Breakfast bars, and Organic Food bars as great, nutrient dense options. (*KF- Read your ingredients*)

YOGURT-COVERED PRETZELS

All snacks exist on a spectrum, and though yogurt-covered pretzels are better than, say, french fries, these nibbles should be treated with caution. Yogurt and yogurt coating are two very different foods – "whereas traditional yogurt is full of calcium, yogurt coating is made of saturated fat, cane syrup, partially hydrogenated palm oil, milk powder, and preservatives," says Cipullo. To avoid consuming a ton of white flour and sugar, Shapiro suggests D.I.Y.-dipping your own version of the treat by dipping whole-wheat pretzels in Greek yogurt.

Fish oil: which contains Omega 3 fatty acids has been shown to help curb appetite, reduce fat storage, enhance overall well-being, and eventually contribute to weight reduction. A good product will contain at least 750 mg of the EPA and DHA, the Omega 3s that give fish oil its benefits per capsule.

Sleep: when we fail to get adequate amounts of sleep, we produce more ghrelin, and as you recall, this hormone is responsible for the feelings of hunger that we have when the stomach is empty. Inadequate sleep produces less leptin (fullness hormone) and can disrupt the insulin, glucose metabolism.

Did you know that salt is used as a substitute for sugar based on the way your taste buds work? Want proof?

Would you ever think to put sugar in tomato soup?

~CLE

Polyphenols: although I hesitate to put this one in this group of options, I think it is important to understand that things like chocolate have a place in weight reduction strategies. The data presented at the

2014 European Atherosclerosis Society Congress showed that food selected because of the high polyphenol content was rather easy for patients to maintain. This particular eating regimen included green tea, coffee, extra virgin olive oil (EVOO), and even dark chocolate notably enhanced glucose metabolism in individuals at high risk for diabetes and cardiovascular disease.

MEDITERRANEAN EATING PRACTICES: shows that an eating regimen complemented with extra-virgin olive oil (EVOO) may cut the risk for developing type 2 diabetes amongst individuals with high risk for cardiovascular disease.

Additional data from the Universitat Rovira i Virgili, in Reus, Spain studies published January 6 in the Annals of Internal Medicine by Jordi Salas-Salvado, MD, Ph.D., and colleagues stated that there is strong evidence that long-term adherence to a Mediterranean cuisine supplemented with EVOO without energy restrictions . . . results in a substantial reduction in the risk for type 2 diabetes among older persons with high cardiovascular risk." The article states, "The Mediterranean diet is high in good fat (30% to 40% of total calories) from vegetable sources such as olive oil and nuts and relatively low in dairy products. The diet also commonly includes sauces with tomato, onions, garlic, and spices and moderate wine consumption."

Struggle is proof
that you have
not yet been conquered...
Fight to be Healthy

~CLE

"Of note, this dietary pattern is palatable and has a high potential for long-term sustainability, with obvious public-health implications for primary prevention of diabetes," the investigators wrote.

I like this study primarily because of the numbers. The study was normed on a quite significant large number of people as well as over a long length of time.

The beneficial cardiovascular effects of the Mediterranean diet are believed to be due to its inclusion of ingredients containing various minerals, polyphenols, and other phytochemicals that combat oxidative stress, inflammation, and insulin resistance, Dr. Salas Salvado and colleagues note.

THE CONCLUSION, summarized in the words of Art Caplan, from the Division of Medical Ethics at the New York University Langone Medical Center in New York is interesting. The reason I say that is because, it seems to reason that doctors must engage in the conversation of overweight, fat, and obesity if there is to be a general change in the weight and healthiness in America's population.

(I have worked with obese doctors who in fact did not tell individuals about their weight as an issue when these patients were having a crisis related to their weight [diabetic hyperglycemia, high blood pressure/ hypertension, etc.])

So, this conclusion is a step in the right direction:

Another weighty notion (pun intended) shared by KF, is that, "…in the US, one of the few countries, where the poorest people tend to be the "fattest in the population. Typically around the world the poorest people are the hungriest and famished making them the smallest of the population"

FOOD FOR THOUGHT:

Single Ingredient Foods

In most cases, this is the best option for eating. These foods tend to be what is called clean in terms of eating. Many of them are raw and freshly grown, and certainly contain less chemicals and unknown treatments.

* Unlimited Eating, especially the raw vegetables, and limited fruit due to sugars.

***

* Multiple Ingredient Foods – *Unrecognizable Items* Decisions, Decisions

Of course none of us know everything . . . so there is never a time when we will know everything about everything we ever consume. However, we should cautiously consider that what we can control we should. And the less of the unknown we put in our bodies the better off we'll be.

* Cautious eating and limited at best

***

* Multiple Ingredient Foods – *Recognizable Items*

There are a couple of rules of thumb when it comes to being good to your body. If you cannot pronounce it, then you shouldn't eat it, and if the ingredient has more than five syllables, then it's probably not going to be good for you to eat and be healthy too.

* Limited as long as you know what you are eating and how it will affect you.

"If we are going to get a handle on the obesity epidemic, then we need to stop saying, 'All you have to do is control your diet,' and somehow manage the responsibility that your genes gives you." Telling people they have a genetic basis for obesity is kind of an excuse or an easy way out.

We must start taking more seriously the dangers that are out in the environment.

For instance, we have to consider saying to each other and to patients and clients, "Hey, those places you drive past that are advertising and marketing 'unhealthy fast food', they're dangerous for you. You might want to avoid them." I think we have to ask people and patients, "How often do you go to these places? How often are you eating there? Do you realize that even if a place has a salad on the menu if you get 3 Big Macs and french fries, it does not matter that a salad is on the menu if you don't order it or even eat it along with the other foods mentioned?"

"We should also think about telling our patients that a lot of fast food promotions and fast-food presence is leading to some of the overweight and obesity problems we see in their kids."

Maybe a better philosophy is to visit and eat at one of the many fast food places as a treat rather than going simply because you have run out of quick and easy meal ideas. It may be easy, but as this study on Mediterranean foods was summarized at NY Langone Medical Center shows fast foods and or not being purposeful in what you eat is dangerous.

In the end, we cannot ever point the finger of blame at our genes or say, hey, exercise some self-control [without providing some support] for people who do not have a controlled eating plan. Let's realize that in a world in which temptation is put out all around us; that is a problem we have to discuss with patients too."

Be present to every moment in your life…you never know when one of your eating moments will be the defining moment in your life…

~CLE

Chapter Four

What's Inside Your Head?

Magic Thought Number One

To help you understand the Two-and-a-Half Magic Thoughts that we've referenced several times already, we have to go inside our mind. We have to see what you see, what you believe, what you say and what it's causing you to do. Some of what you have thought has been good and maybe even beneficial for you . . . (proof: you're still alive). Other thoughts – and one in particular that I am aware of, has probably been the most destructive and harmful to you and even the cause of most of your setbacks. I believe the wait is over. At the least, we'll remove it at the roots and set you free to use the other one and a half thoughts to propel you toward your achievement and victory. How do I know, you might ask (assuming I'm not presumptuous). Well, you're reading this book for one which tells me you want something you may not have at the moment: your ultimate healthiness.

It is important to stake the rest of your reading and the work you will do as you read, in an absolute moment of honesty. You know better than anyone else what you have thought in private. You, more than anyone else knows what you have thought and even said when you have seriously tried in the past to reduce your weight. And only you know what you have thought and said when you have tried to exercise to reduce your weight and it hurt, felt awful, and frustrated you because you had no results. So let's get at these thoughts and really look at them to see if we even want to keep them for future use.

To begin, I'd like for you to list at least five of your thoughts, concerns, and frustrations you've had while working to get rid of unwanted weight and fat – this battle may have raged on for years and years, and you've thought many things (maybe more things than you care to remember.)

She is braver who overcomes her fear of sharing her inner thoughts than she who overcomes her rivals:

For the hardest conquest is the conquest over one's self

~CLE

Now, as you think back through time, I want you only to remember those thoughts or comments that were strong enough to create emotion in you. (For instance: "this is too tough," "nothing works," and "that was a complete waste of money" [and it might have been], or even "I give up" or that gut wrenching throat sound that sounds like UGHHHH)!

Go ahead and list at least five of these thoughts now. *(Consider doing this on a disposable piece of paper and finish reading until you are prompted to stop and close the book or until an overwhelming thought comes to mind and you have to write it down now.)*

Want to know how your future will be five years from now; listen to what you're saying about yourself, and your life in the present moment.

~ CLE

So what was the purpose of writing down these thoughts even before you understand these two-and-a-half thoughts?

Because, like building a house, you wouldn't place new wood or concrete on top of a broken, dilapidated, condemned structure. To maximize the benefits of the two-and-a-half magic thoughts we have to root out the detrimental thoughts that you have programmed into your brain's everyday thinking. It is largely your foundation or your beliefs that have allowed these thoughts to become your everyday thinking. So, that's where we need to begin our cleansing work.

And for the clearing-cleansing process to really provide the greatest results, you must do this exercise of writing these thoughts down with every bit of integrity and honesty you have in you. If you commit to doing this simple, easy, and harmless exercise the way I have asked you, you will all but guarantee your results. So, begin now with the intention of finishing.

I can safely believe that you've also said some things about fat and your personal condition: things like,

- "well it's OK, everybody has a little fat,"
- "it's not that bad,"
- "I'll get rid of it someday,"
- "I'll just wear looser clothes or the tent dress that covers everything,"
- "it's just baby-fat,"
- . . . the guys' favorite, "I'll start working out when . . .,"
- "we all gotta die from something."

– cause I said some of these things too. I'm not sure I should have been surprised however, when I found out that many of the fat people around me did too when I asked them about it. (Seven years of surveys, interviews and interactions with over 80% of the people interviewed agreeing to having had similar thoughts).

Never let settling for good be an excuse to keep you from great. Good enough is often an enemy to being great.

~CLE

How have you portrayed or even rationalized being overweight? We've all done it. We look in the mirror and suck in our tummies or turn certain ways to see our "best" angles (standing tall with our back straight). Then, we say to ourselves, "That's not so bad," or "I look good to me, and that's all that matters." Or maybe even the proverbial, "I've tried everything," "I'll just get the surgery when I can afford it," and on and on, over and over again. Of course, when we say these things over a period of time, our brains pick up on the pattern, believing that what we're saying even if internally, is what we want. Then our brain creates a neural blueprint that allows us to think these thoughts more easily and more often, such that, we end up believing it over time.

And because your unconscious now, does not know the difference between what is real and what is not, it will only know what you tell it. Each time you start any one of these types of thoughts you've had in the past now, your brain fires up the old pattern you're used to and the pattern gets repeated. It is an auto-pilot behavior that automatically opens mental files, which then completes the sequence of other thoughts allowing you to rationalize being overweight over time. This ongoing cycle plays back thoughts and language patterns that say the same things over and over again – "that we are just fine" and "it'll be OK." And the truth of the matter is that we consciously know that we are not "just fine or OK." If we were, we would not be looking in the mirror at our bodies and having these thoughts in the first place. The virtue of truth is if we were totally honest, with all of the information available, then we'd admit that we are slowly contributing to our death.

Yes, I did say that. If you are obese and this part of your life is out of control and you have health-related symptoms, then you are what is called "Morbid Obese." The field of medicine, your insurance company, the Center for Disease Control, The Surgeon General, The National Institute of Health and a host of other organizations, all believe you being overweight is going to contribute to your death; sooner rather than later.

The insurance company believes it so much that they are charging you more, whether you know it or not, covering your absolute expenses related to death. Other medical/health insurance and life insurers make you pay for being this way too. Of course most of us don't like parting with our money and spending it on issues we can easily change.

So, it is Urgent and Important that we find the cause of your complacency, rationalization, and irrational hope of a miracle that you'll wake up one day and it will all be different with nothing else having happened. Know that the idea of wishful thinking without any effort at all will not change your life, but you can: and, you can begin the change process right now!

The past can never be altered.
The future, however is yours and yours alone to control and even change now.
~ CLE

The miracle wish won't end up the way we imagine it might if you were so inclined to think it, at least not as a result of the way we have thought to do things in the past.

Once you root out these detrimental thoughts and learn the Two-and-a-Half Magic Thoughts, then you will in fact undoubtedly wake up one morning and before you even get out of the bed or off the couch or wherever you've slept, you'll know that your thinking is different. You will have become a new someone, (the particular person) you must be – the only one who can easily make your dreams and desires come true.

<u>DO THIS</u>:
Spend a few minutes now, allowing yourself to think about the things you've thought and said. At first, it will seem like popcorn when it's first popping: the thoughts you've had will almost overwhelm you. You'll think about all kinds of things you've said and thought.

(WRITE THEM DOWN on a disposable piece of paper as they come, and use as many pieces of paper as it takes.) The idea here is to get them out of your head and onto the paper – this is simply a representation or an external place for them to reside. Anywhere is better than keeping them inside of your head.

CLOSE THE BOOK AND WORK
ON *THIS EXERCISE NOW!*

DO NOT CONTINUE READING
UNTIL YOU HAVE FINSIHED.

It's only too late
when you have taken your last breath.
That's not the case so,
let's get moving towards
CHANGE NOW!
~CLE

Remember, the idea of wishful thinking without any effort at all will not change your life, but *you* can: and, you can begin the change process now!

Once you root out these detrimental thoughts and learn the Two-and-a-Half Magic Thoughts, you have more than a fighting chance of actually winning the battle you've been fighting. It will allow you to actually wake up to and know that *you are different.* You will have become a new someone, the particular person you want to be – the only person who makes your dreams and hopes become reality.

The actions you take are the best indicators of what you really think
Act Now-
Do Something
~CLE

Now, because you've diligently completed the task of cleaning out some of the thoughts that stop you from getting the results you want, we can easily move on to the real thrill of this book. We'll also begin to get rid of those thoughts forever, right now.

First, can I share a brief story with you?

I once knew of a young man about the age of 12-13. The young man was a good kid but sometimes he would be swayed by other kids. You know how kids often sway other kids, don't you?

This young man had a good friend by the name of Jerry. Jerry's dad owned a pool hall. This place absolutely fascinated the young boy and Jerry. They would spend every possible moment there, watching how men played, joking around and drinking.

Now Jerry's dad was not always as honest as he could be. He was noted for taking the bottom portion of each liquor bottle and pouring several blends together creating a "house blend."

Jerry and the young man would sneak into Jerry's dad's barn and find these small portions of leftover liquor. You guessed it: they drank some of them quite often, and sometimes they drank too much –way too much. The boys thought they had a good thing going and a great big secret indulging themselves when no one was looking. But once, they had just a little too much of the house blend – more than their bodies could handle and mom found out ("cause it's hard to fake gluttony and sobriety when it comes right down to it.") Of course, being more than just a little on the tipsy side the young man gave mom way more information than she asked for. The young man had a moment of honesty-freedom. He was able to let go, confess and free himself from the guilt, shame and the hiding of the past).

Mom sat waiting for dad, and together they talked about the problem facing their son. Both of them loved their child more than anything else in life. They came to this conclusion about their child's secret: if things stayed the same there would be a loss of control, and moreover, they would lose him.

So, they placed their house up for sale and soon after that, sold it. Now the difficult choice began. "To where do we move?" They found a small 40-acre hillside farm several miles from the city, with the nearest neighbor more than 2 miles away.

Here was a young man from the city who had been surrounded by the things he loves, his friends, the pool hall, the house blend, and of course his best friend, Jerry. The young man awoke one day and realized he was alone for the first time. He hated the stillness of the new place. He missed the sounds of the city.

He missed the foul tobacco smell of the pool hall as well as the occasional snack from the bar's food supply. And not hearing the sounds of his friends' voices was almost more than he could bear.

The young man's parents thought they had found the solution to their problem, but realized they had only found a different set of problems. The young man now expressed his anger at being alone in terms that caused his parents to sometimes question their wisdom.

One day the young man was on the hillside just walking and kicking the rocks along the hillside – a hillside that was barren of everything but rock and cactus. He was disgusted with life. He could feel his rage inside him rise with each step. He began to kick the stones that lay on top of the ground with an unfocused fury. He would kick the rock and then take a deep breath and yell a few colorful words at the silence of the world.

On the next kick, the young man made, a strange thing appeared. Under the stone and hidden from the midday sun rays, appeared a scorpion. A huge dirt-colored scorpion appeared from under the rock. This scorpion was so big to the young man that it frightened him for a moment. Then he thought, "Jerry has never seen a scorpion and if I catch it, maybe Mom will take me to see Jerry."

The young man began thinking of ways to catch the scorpion. He would go around to the right, and the scorpion would turn with him. Each time he turned the scorpion would reach out trying to attack with its massive claw, trying to sting you with its powerful tale of poison and anxiety. This *went on for a long time* going left and then right and *getting faster even now.* Suddenly the young man thought of using his tee shirt. He took his shirt off and threw it over the scorpion. The scorpion grabbed hold of the shirt. The young man then picked up the shirt as the scorpion held on and violently stuck the shirt with its poisonous tail.

The young man ran up the hill straight to his house yelling, "Mom, Mom, Mom look what I've got!" Of course, Mom simply yelled at the top of her lungs capacity, "Get that thing out of this house!" The young man kept saying, "Mom I have to save this scorpion so I can take it to Jerry's." Mom kept saying no and the young man would repeat himself.

Mom finally became fearful that the scorpion would turn loose of the shirt and then she would really have a problem. She saw a gallon, sun tea jar on the counter and quickly opened the lid and told her son to shake the scorpion loose into the iced tea jar. On the third shake, the scorpion hit the bottom of the jar, "tink" with a crisp sound of insect armor meeting glass.

The scorpion would go around the bottom of the glass, and you could hear the sounds of the scraping and clicking of its tail against the glass. Mom yelled at her son to "get it out of the house now!"

Of course, the young man saw something different. "Mom, we have to take this to Jerry. Jerry has never seen a scorpion before. It would be so neat for Jerry to have this to take to school."

The young man's mother got stronger in her response with each request to take the scorpion to see Jerry. Finally, he gave up for the day and took the jar to his room.

Do you think the young man gave up on his mission to take the scorpion to Jerry? (. . . isn't that the way our desire is sometimes: persistent?)

Of course not – he was just like every other kid wanting to see a friend. He would be tugging at his mom's pant leg each time he got a chance. Finally a couple of weeks later she reluctantly said, "I have to go into town so you can get that scorpion and take it to Jerry's. You can't stay long, but at least you can leave the scorpion with him."

The young man ran into his room and grabbed the jar. He returns to the kitchen sad and dejected.

His mother looks at him dragging his feet and immediately knows that something is terribly wrong. Then she sees the scorpion is dead in the jar and sees the tears on her son's cheeks.

She tells her son, "Listen I have a great idea." She gets a small jar out and places the dead scorpion into the container. She then fills the container with alcohol. "Look here son, the scorpion is now harmless in the jar and will be safe for Jerry to take to school. And you know this scorpion will last a long time now." She could see that her son accepted the solution.

After a long day of errands and shopping, they finally are ready to go to Jerry's house. The young man can hardly wait to show the scorpion to his friend Jerry. It's something that Jerry has never seen, and he saw it first and caught it too. He could not sit still in his seat in the car and counted down the houses until finally, they arrived at Jerry's.

The young man immediately ran up to the door and pounded, but no one answered. He rang the doorbell and beat the door again. Still, no one came.

Mom could see the hurt on her son's face and thought of a solution. When the young man returned to the car, they took the groceries out of one of the bags. She wrote, "SCORPION" in bold, black ink on the bag, placed the jar in the bag and simply rolled the bag up.

"Here, go place this on the porch, and when they get home, they will see the surprise." So they drove off leaving the scorpion in the bag on the front porch.

Jerry and his mom got back from their errands and shopping and began the process of taking the groceries into the house. Jerry's mom was walking up to the porch when she saw the bag. She was curious, and suddenly she became frightened. She saw the bold word scorpion. She had seen a special on TV about scorpions and knew she was in danger. She knew that the scorpion could easily stick its stinger through the paper bag and poison them.

Jerry's mother grabbed him and told him to carry all of the groceries into the back door of the house. Jerry's dad would have to deal with the scorpion in a few days. "If we go thru the back door of the house and never confront it," she thought, "we will be safe."

So they left the bag on the porch. On Saturday morning, Jerry's mother looked out the window and saw a small blond-haired boy. She saw him looking at the bag on the porch. Immediately she had a mental picture of this boy being stung by the scorpion and lying on the grass gasping for air. She knew she would be sued and become so poor that they would have nothing. All because of this stupid scorpion in a bag on the front porch and she didn't even know where it came from.

She ran through the house, threw open the door and discovered she was too late. The blond boy had already opened up the bag. He was holding up this small jar with something dead in the bottom. She was so relieved!

Then she thought. "Wow, when I thought the dead scorpion was alive, rolled up in that bag, it had so much power over me. Its power made me go thru the back door of my home, totally unwilling to confront it. I totally changed my behavior and who I am in this secure environment of my house."

...And that's the way our thoughts work, almost like secrets. As long as we keep our secrets rolled up in a bag or inside of us, they have so much power over us. It's only when we allow our thoughts and the secrets we keep about our health, weight and our perception of ourselves to come out into the open and we expose them to see what they really are; just a dead scorpion. Then we can enter our life through the front door and really live. Allowing others to be an active part of what is going on in our world by helping us to see where our weaknesses are, gives us encouragement and accountability, to be our best. That will help us to be and do better in our efforts and attempts to be healthy.

So many secrets, and so much hidden inside means there is no light to help us see what "it" really is and that "it" has no real effect or power over us (unless we interpret it to). I wonder if it is possible for this shedding of light on our thoughts to lessen the weight of my own secrets, so that when it happens, I will not be able to contain my laughter at such a silly thing and the way I have acted for so long. (Stressing out, secretly eating to assuage my discomforts, uncertainties, insecurities, disappointments, and even eating because I was thirsty or worse, "bored.")

And now, you can finish your brief assignment. As a point of reference, I do know personally what it is like to keep what I feel and think inside and never let it out. I also know the toll it took on my life and my well-being when I did that. If you have not completed the exercise, you must *do it now.*

No Human is a solo-element of life- We all will affect and be affected by someone else

~CLE

The sky is not the limit it is simply a view. Live with no limits and impose your purpose on your life instead of imposing limits.

~CLE

The most effective way to insure the value of your future is to confront the present courageously and constructively.

ACT NOW![3]

~Rollo May

Chapter Five

The Truth and the Language We Use to Express It

Magic Thought Number Two

Now let's begin with the most important factor no one has ever told you. When you get it now, your life will never be the same. It will prompt your subconscious to release new chemicals and an incredible active set of habitual thoughts into your body and your life.

This is huge, big, massive, large and incredible. It is fundamental to every bit of success in weight reduction and really letting the healthier, slender you live, live and live! If you have ever said to yourself or to others in the past that "it's hard to experience weight reduction or, that you've had no success in getting over the hump (there just seemed to be a point where you could not get it going) oh, and don't forget "I really didn't have the time to exercise" or I felt like I was trapped," your release is about to be revealed to you in ONE simple thought.

I promise that the stark reality of your success no matter what else you do, like seeing yourself exercising, walking, moving your arms, eating less and moving more in general, all, fundamentally depend on how you visualize yourself through this next section. Are you ready? I mean are you really ready for the truth of the whole matter?

Well, if *you are* really *ready now*, then let's go inside your mind to get at the truth and nothing but the truth, for it is that which sets you free.

As you can begin to read further you can relax even more, knowing that for the rest of your life nothing can stop you from reaching your dream of being smaller and healthy. Now, you will notice that what you will read next will have already caused you to feel less stressed about dropping the weight forever.

First, the previous battle you've had and already won has everything to do with "Weight Loss" itself and the challenges it has brought you. AS HELPFUL AS IT MIGHT HAVE SEEMED THEN – AS COMMON

...and the truth shall set you free.[4]

~Adapted from John 3:2 NIV

AS IT IS TO SAY AND THE FACT THAT EVERYONE IS SAYING IT, and as bizarre as it will be, to finally understand

WEIGHT LOSS DOES NOT EXIST

I can only imagine what you're thinking at this point; "There's been millions and even billions of dollars spent on weight loss programs, supplements, machinery, gadgets, fads, sweat aids, vibrating machines, drinks, prescriptions, creams, potions, diets, advice, and medical attention from people like "Dr. Oz" (and I mean that kindly as a personal friend in the nicest way possible.) There's even lotions, shakes videos, hypnosis, and surgical procedures all in the name of *weight loss!* So, how can there be no such thing?"

Well, the first clue is that you are reading this book as opposed to enjoying your desired results. If the elusive weight loss phenomenon existed as does air, cups, and sidewalks, the general population would have ready access to it and would be able to put their hands on it with demonstrated results. The second is that you are probably part of the 58% of the general population looking to reduce their body fat and live a healthy slender life (and although you will soon be getting that) you have not in the past gotten the results you were after. You can however, begin right now! As a result of what you learn here, you will be able to put into action a whole new approach to living healthier.

As you read this, inside, you can already begin to feel a change as you relax in knowing the truth. If you are over 7 years old, then you have already experienced why *there is no such thing as weight loss.* Yet, you have allowed your mind to determine that it does exist, based on word patterning, linguistic acceptance and social agreement, (Isopraxism) – weight loss being a term that has had no real value for you or anybody else as it relates to getting healthier weight results.

Now what does all this mean? Simply this: Society has determined how you got your results and you bought into it either consciously or unconsciously. As a result, you chose to use the language, methods and behaviors that went along with their approaches and most often got their results. Let me explain it to you.

Over your lifetime you have undoubtedly lost thousands of things. I hear you chuckling. I mean some of us have even lost our cars for Pete's sake. (Or maybe I should speak for my own sake.) I lost my car while in Greenwich Village NY once, while out on a date, and oh my goodness, the stress! I've even heard of someone who actually called the police and filed a stolen vehicle report at a local home improvement store because his truck was stolen and he had looked for 30 minutes. After calling his wife he was told his truck was in the driveway and that he had driven her car to the store. My point is simply that we have moments when we lose things from our present memory banks. Haven't you?

There is one thing stranger than all the world and that is an idea whose time has come![5]

~ Victor Hugo

Now, I already know the answer is yes to many of the following questions, yet I'm going to ask them for your benefit in helping you understand why there is no such thing as weight loss. "Have you ever lost your keys?" "Have you ever lost a remote control?" Or how about the cordless phone, a shoe, an earring, pen, glasses, watch, tools, rings, teeth (false ones too), a gadget, socks, cell phone, cosmetics, contact lenses, books, a jacket, CD, files, a button, umbrella, money, a purse, credit card, wallet, shopping bag full of the groceries you were supposed to bring home, documents—like social security cards, your license, an important letter or piece of paper or items that you thought were in a box when you moved from one house to another, cell phone, kids(?) or how about the fact that some us of have lost our minds and still haven't found them (lol)? And I can hear some of you saying now, "I didn't lose any of those things, I simply misplaced them or did not remember where they were."

We act only on what we believe . . .
Change what you believe and you will always get a different result!
~CLE

Ok, c'mon now, call a spade a spade and enough with the splitting of semantic hairs. The Bottom Line Is That YOU LOST IT! That's the truth of the matter.

And as you have grown older, the number of things you've lost has grown exponentially. And, every single time you have ever lost anything, what have you done?

What have you always done and what will you continue to do in the future when you lose anyone of the things above. What do you do automatically?

Answer ____

Because you are doing this with complete integrity and honesty your answer above is most likely, *"I try to find it."* Certainly, when you have lost really valuable things *you looked for them,* didn't you? OF COURSE you did! No one had to tell you, ask you or get you motivated to do it. You automatically begin to search for the items. They all are valuable to you in some way. You wanted things to be the same before you lost the keys or whatever it was. That is the way we are created; to maintain some sense of normalcy or sameness in our lives.

Your brain (hypothalamus) has developed one of the most incredible automatic habits of keeping you "normal" by stabilizing everything you choose to control in your life. Anything you lose that has become a part of how you function, no matter if for just a brief time, your brain tries to keep track of it, to keep it the same, to normalize it. So, whenever you lose anything, your brain kicks into autopilot and seeks to find what's lost to keep things "normal."

Now think about this . . .

Above all else in life is the need to experience things that make us happy. Often we have to fight with ourselves to keep our lives balanced when things change and they will.

~CLE

Think about how painful it is when someone close to you dies. Think about the feeling of emptiness you experience when you LOSE a loved one. Perhaps the feelings are close or equal to when you lose a friendship, relationship or even a family pet. There is a very serious pain in our minds when we lose things.

And because your brain is created for and programmed to *avoid pain and seek pleasure* it will resist the loss of anything. Why do you think we have so much distress when it comes to even just thinking about what will happen when we lose things? Literally, most of what is considered "worry" is just our minds thinking about potential losses. LOSS, LOSS, LOSS = PAIN, PAIN, PAIN. Are you starting to see why you must reprogram your brain away from thinking and saying WEIGHT-LOSS when it comes to changing your weight? WHERE THERE IS "WEIGHT-LOSS," there is PAIN, with a Capital P along with many of pains' relatives, mostly in our minds, unconsciously.

So, we must understand this FACT first – it's the only way that you can ever get rid of the weight permanently. The healthy, slender, POWERFUL you is ready and so now you must know forever that THERE IS NO SUCH THING AS WEIGHT LOSS because the moment you actually might "lose" 5, 10 pounds your brain is on auto-pilot looking to find anything that you lose. Ever heard of yo-yo dieting? Ever heard of gaining it all back? Ever heard of fluctuating, bouncing or even the statement, "I go between _____ and _____"?

It's already occurred in your life a hundred thousand times over and is so routine in your unconscious mind that it is impossible to keep your brain from doing it, until now. The unwanted weight seems to be lurking right around every corner. The moment you brag, celebrate or even confidently reward yourself, the quicker the scale says you've started gaining it back. And then you find over the next few days that "fluctuation thing" happening.

Take time to deliberate, but when the time for action arrives, STOP thinking and Do It![6]

~Andrew Jackson

Your body seems to revolt and you feel bloated or even just fat (in your stomach particularly). Then, you get frustrated trying to figure out what you ate and how this could be happening. Now of course, if you are on pace in your weight reduction and then all of a sudden things come to a screeching halt and seems to be moving in reverse – you conscientiously sound the inner alarm and defensively try to preserve what you've been able to achieve. You stop eating, afraid to eat anything, not wanting to fully reverse the course which your body has a natural reaction to as well (your body thinks you're starving it and in order to survive, holds on to – *fat* as a means of providing fuel, nutrition insulation, etc.) Finally, when it's too overpowering, or the hunger is too much, you eat and slowly find yourself in a lot of instances right back or close to where you started.

Nonetheless, your brain is automatically triggered to find a way to get back to "NORMAL" and "gain" some if not all of that weight back onto your body frame. Then, you'll find that there is a battle between your mind and body as it becomes a conscious struggle to achieve your desired results. The frustration occupies your time, your mind and your conversation (with others and self). You definitely want the change but the effort just seems to beat you up, over and over again. Unfortunately, the first set back is not knowing that the beginning of any newly desired behavior (especially weight reduction efforts) starts with the battle of six inches. It is critical, urgent and important to your results and your health to know that these six inches are not in your waist, tummy or even your thighs. It is the space between your ears.

Motivation will almost always win over mere ability.[7]

~ Norman Augustine

You would literally have to double the calorie burn (exercise) every day (that is if you eat 2000 calories daily you would have to burn nearly 4000 calories) to *"trick"* your brain into the physical habit of being able to *"lose"* weight based on how our brains respond to losing anything. For this type of process to work, it would have to solely be a factor of your physiology and barely anything to do with your thinking for you to really "lose" the weight you desire.

First, know that you must get inside your unconscious patterns (automatically triggered thoughts) rather than find a program, a machine or a diet. Changing your mind must be the beginning of your transformation. This is the only way to get your brain to produce new chemical patterns, which link with new thinking patterns and ultimately new behavioral patterns. This will free you from any form of excess weight and unhealthy eating behaviors.

Secondly, (let's be as practical and as simple as we can possibly be) GET RID OF THE TERMS "LOSING WEIGHT", "Weight Loss", "Lose Weight", and even "Diet" for that matter. Do not limit what you get rid of; just remove all of the terms, statements, and thoughts you have had in the past that you now know are detrimental to your desires and healthiness.

INSTEAD, begin now – stating the results you want. For example you find yourself carrying 25, 50, 100 or 200 pounds or more than you want to, then state what it is that you want and how you want to be. "I will be 140 pounds." "I must be 140 pounds." "I can certainly see myself with a body carrying 160 pounds." "You know, 200 pounds feels great." "Today my body and mind will create the conditions and appropriate desires to form and shape my body to 138 pounds." We will work on this a little later, but for now we must finish getting rid of the detrimental thoughts.

Be aware that you will always end up traveling in the direction you are heading. For all of us, there is always room in our lives for thinking that we can do the things that have been our biggest challenges, for pushing the limits, and really imagining the possibilities of who you were created to be.

"Life is a dream, realize it.
Life is a challenge, meet it.
Life is a duty, complete it.
Life has sorrow, overcome it.
Life is an adventure, dare to live it.
Life is good, fight for it."[8]

~ Anonymous

If you have been challenged with being out of shape (whatever that means to you), carrying more weight than you want to, temporarily unable to enjoy a healthy, fit lifestyle and desiring to let the real (deep down inside) you out, then your brief journey has finally begun. Congratulations! You have overcome the most difficult part of weight reduction, weight control, healthy living, being physically fit and even being able to actually visualize mentally what you will look like in your future now. By understanding the language of your mind (the unconscious automatic triggers) and the habits that show up in your conscious day-to-day behavior you can have the results you are after.

If your past language patterns have had you saying things that include any of the previous weight loss terms, you have unfortunately been engaged in a repetitive cycle of up and down, up and down (regardless of what you've tried). And because you are beginning to understand how your brain operates – YOUR BRAIN IS DESIGNED TO DO AND OR TO CREATE WHATEVER YOU TELL IT – thus you can see why it has been such a struggle until now.

No more weight loss – it simply does not exist. It cannot exist because of the way we have developed our lives, our thinking and our automated unconscious behavior. It cannot exist because of the way our brains perceive any type of LOSS. The truth is that we will try, often desperately, to find, have and cherish anything we lose. Weight is the same. We simply cannot lose it. Not now – not ever!

Bottom Line: Stop thinking "weight loss." How? Stop saying it! Stop writing it in your diary or your journal! Delete it from your vocabulary! Stop thinking it when you look at yourself in the mirror! Find another reason for going to the gym, exercising, walking, etc. STOP talking about losing weight! Eliminate it from your conversation with others and by God, STOP believing it exists, because it doesn't, and *do it now* for Heaven's sake!

Change is one of the most difficult things we do as humans. Yet we have so many examples of the benefits of change.

For instance, flowers, butterflies, being able to feed ourselves versus being fed as a baby, night and day, etc. . . . When change has the potential to change you for the better, no matter how tough it is. . . .

You must purpose that you want to change and that you must change – so that you will change, now!

Always remember- Weight Loss does not exist!

ALTERNATIVES to the term weight loss:

- Dropping the weight*
- Take off the weight*
- Get rid of the weight (unwanted pounds)*

- Getting healthier
- Creating a healthier me
- Reshaping me
- Getting fit and healthy
- Inspired to be my best me
- Getting rid of the junk on my body
- Cleaning my body
- Cleansing my mind and body of the weight holding me back from life

The terms highlighted above are there because of their subconscious power. Many times in the past you have gotten rid of things never to see them again and many of those things you threw away and never thought twice about seeing them and or wanting anything to do with them again. For most of us we take off clothing on a daily basis and when those clothes are off and we are done with them we place them in their proper place like the closet or the dirty laundry and forget about them (we're simply done with them). As mentioned in one of the quotes often we have to drop the rope we hold onto so desperately – as it drags us into the past lest we suffer burns to our hands – Simply dropping it and letting it go is a great way to have your mind designed to let it go forever.

Chapter Six

Creating a New You

One Half Magic Thought

You have already learned the most important of beliefs related to changing your weight. This change is that there is no "weight loss." You've already shown by completing the previous exercises and demonstrated by your ongoing reading here, that you are serious about being rid of awful beliefs that support awful thinking. You have said perhaps without speaking that you will use language that points your mind in the direction you want to go. Always remember, that in addition to what you have already established this is really about your health and not just your weight. This way and only this way will your mind be able to undo the stagnant results you have been getting . . . and . . . because there is no such thing as real weight-loss, we get to move on almost effortlessly.

For many of us, we've heard so much about weight, we've seen so much about preferred body types, about being fit, about how thin is in, about exercise, about supplements, diets, exercise machines about things that melt the fat away, about miracle pills and the like. Just who are the people behind all of this stuff and who is it that they think we are?

The truth is that many of the producers of these trends, products and images are people who really have no valid clue about "weight".

In many cases they know nothing about being in shape, fitness and in many cases are unhealthy themselves. (I will admit however, that they are fairly good business, marketing and public relations strategists). Who They Think We Are, Is Different, because this is where they've been winning big-time over the last half of the century. In many cases their desires become yours.

Your dreams will be just that,
dreams, unless
you act.
You can act slow or you can
act fast.
The choice is yours.
Understand, however, that
LIFE
WILL NOT WAIT for you to
decide.
~CLE

This is not just my opinion. I'm sure you have seen many of these people defending their products and selling manipulation to the public on TV, in the mall, on the radio, etc. In some cases many of these trends and products have some merit. Unfortunately, the emphasis is clearly in the most inappropriate places.

I mean we've all heard sayings that many of us have repeated and some us have bought into, (i.e. an apple a day keeps the doctor away, starve a cold – feed a fever, come in out of the rain or you'll catch your death from a cold, or even a cold draft will give you a sore throat.) and for most of us this is how we develop our thoughts about what is really important to our bodies and our healthiness. We are often shaped by what we hear constantly and what we see as well. We are told that being fit is the way our healthiness is demonstrated in our culture.

The truth is that life is never about being physically fit. If that were true then world class marathon runners would never drop dead in the middle of a race, and people like Arthur Ashe would not have keeled over with a heart attack while teaching a tennis clinic; the game he trained his physical heart to respond to and his mental-heart to love for 20 plus years. Did you know the average life span of a doctor is 58 years of age? Apparently, they haven't learned to scrub their brain either of the daily bombardment of incorrect and uninspiring messages we all tend to get. If I may be so bold without offending any reader . . . (just don't tell them I said this—) "they eat some of the same "crap" as normal people when they are stressed, depressed, undisciplined, etc. and yes, many of them are a bit obese as a result." But that's not the point, which is, that many of them have not figured out that Fit and Thin Does Not Equal Healthy, although many of them know this intuitively through their practice of medicine. . . . They in fact know what healthy is and what it looks like and it still often evades them too.

In the effort to really extend your life, your well-being, and your ability to *feel great mentally, physically, emotionally, socially and often spiritually,* sometimes *for no reason at all* we have to look at something completely different.

It is my opinion that sometimes we are motivated by fear . . . and sometimes, surprisingly, someone comes along with something to share with us, that interestingly is supposed to and just might resolve the thing we are fearful of. Consider carefully and proceed with the greatest of urgency once you decide.

~CLE

HEALTH – the importance of your physical health is the most critical element you can undertake in reducing your weight. No matter your income, success levels, relationships or even your livelihood – NOTHING ELSE MATTERS IF YOU DO NOT HAVE YOUR HEALTH.

Hopefully the statement above makes sense to you. If it doesn't, please take time to think about someone you may know, who has some severe health challenges and either observe the changes they have had to make to accommodate their life or ask them, what it is they want most, now that they are facing the challenge. I'm sure somehow, it will lead right back to the quality of their health. I only know this because I have asked the question hundreds of times and have gotten the same answer. As well, if you were to ask anyone who has survived a heart attack, stroke or severe injury and has resumed a somewhat normal lifestyle, if they are happy they have a second chance, I'm sure 9 out of ten will enthusiastically tell you "yes". This too I have asked.

You will be challenged to be able to enjoy much of anything in this life if you do not have your health. Think about it. If because of things you have ingested, (unhealthily) or because of things you did not correct or attend to while you still have healthy thinking faculties and physiological capabilities – you end up confined, incapacitated, unable, amputated, and or on machines to support your life functions; Would you really – Could you really or will that be the time when you really enjoy your family, enjoy the laughter with friends, enjoy children playing, celebrations, traveling, walking, trees, food, the beach, mountains, the outdoors, or any other of God's creations?

Perhaps you're starting to see how important your health really is.

If you have been obsessed with being fit or you go to the gym and they have you focus on being fit and not being healthy, STOP IMMEDIATELY and find the balance of your efforts with healthiness.

I mean after all, what good would it be if your gas-car looked great on the outside and you put diesel "gas" into the fuel system and then smashed many of the items under the hood with a sledgehammer?

The system ran great and looked great but it was destined to fall apart, fail miserably and have severe costs associated with it eventually. This is different than a car that runs for 85 years and no matter how much you restore it, the parts just wear out. Being fit guarantees you the system looks great and will help (minutely if any) with the internal systems functionality.

In so many instances a large number of us in fact know what to do – It's the execution part that is so elusive.

(*ACT NOW BEFORE YOU* HAVE A CHANCE TO *THINK* YOURSELF OUT OF IT!)

Healthiness includes what you put in to the system. Putting more of what the body is made out of – water (8 – 10 glasses daily), eating as cleanly as possible, making sure you're getting the right balance of nutrients (vitamins, minerals, carbohydrates, proteins, fat and yes, water), and reducing your body fat, always contributes to the system looking great, requires a tiny bit of effort, a dash of commitment, and a never ending cup of want to. This type of effort when given, should, simply be because you can do it. If you are able to do some aerobic movement or even anaerobic movement it will be your key to eliminating waste, fat and other toxins from your body and create a smooth running engine. In simple, if you can move, move, if you cannot, then it has to be done with caloric intake in a way that allows your body to do one of two things explained next.

The human body is AMAZING. I mean really amazing. Everything you put into your body registers in your brain. Your screening mechanisms extract useable nutrients and make every attempt to do away with items in the body that are not useable. Let me explain it another way. Your body either ASSIMILATES what you put in your body or ELIMINATES it. (Of course if it cannot do either, the potential for other kinds of problems is pretty high – so, be careful what you are putting in your body.)

From this point forward in this book and in life it is important to think about your efforts to reduce your weight in terms of being healthy (period). Think about what you're putting in your body in terms of whether it will be assimilated or eliminated. When you choose to say to yourself (and I will give you the reasons why you want to now) – "I CHOOSE TO BE HEALTHY . . ." you have started to understand how these 2 ½ thoughts work together – your beliefs (who you are / what you think-[no weight loss]) and language (what you say and how you act) are key elements.

"Life is like riding a bicycle. To keep your balance, you must keep moving."[9]

~ Paraphrase from Albert Einstein

What is it to be healthy to live fully anyway; moreover, what is health itself? Here are a couple of definitions that you'll want to consider so that you adopt them into your new thought patterns now.

ENCYCLOPEDIA OF NATURAL MEDICINE: health is the result of individual responsibility . . . choosing healthy alternatives over non-healthy.

WORLD HEALTH ORGANIZATION: health is a state of complete physical, mental or social well-being and not merely the absence of disease or infirmity.

RESILIENCY INC: The ability to adapt to stimuli, including infection, circumstance, stress etc.

> Ultimately, healthiness is the epitome of human fulfillment and productivity as well as the best quality of life possible. That is what it all boils down to. Unfortunately, many of us have disregarded it and have to pay the price to have it repaired, rejuvenated and jumpstarted or pay the price of being disabled or even death when the there are no other options available.

You've gotta dance like there's nobody watching, Love like you'll never be hurt, sing like there's nobody listening and live like it's heaven on earth.[10]

~William W. Purkey

The truth is that your efforts must never be about just reducing your weight – it must be about (BE)ING A HEALTHIER YOU Now! That is truth.

So, you must retain and use the two thoughts we have covered (using the appropriate language to express what you want so that your beliefs line up with your capability [healthy vs. weight loss], ridding yourself of negative thought patterns, understanding what's really important in changing your weight, etc.) making a shift in the way you feel about yourself and what you tell yourself you want to be (all prompted by your language and beliefs). Slender, slimmer is good but it is not the end all – be all, when it's all said and done. It can leave you deficient as you find yourself reducing your weight now. To get the complete package you must use your mind's eye, creativity and some re-imaging to see yourself the way you can be and you have got to be innovative in how you maintain your thinking about this image.

"All truth goes through three steps:

First it is ridiculed, Second, it is violently opposed.

Finally, it is accepted as self-evident . . . as if it always existed."[11]

~Shoppenhauer

How about a moment of honesty – a moment of freedom (time to let go, confess and be free from the guilt, shame and hiding of the past). In the past you already knew that your thoughts and what you believed was possible for you, weren't strong enough to keep your mind focused or strong enough to provide you the motivation, incentive or reinforcement to get into action. It wasn't strong enough to do what was necessary to help you, be the- you, you really want to be.

Additionally, the necessities for getting yourself slender and keeping yourself slender just weren't there. It was because the image was missing some of the key elements of being healthy. It was just an image of a physical you and incomplete without a health oriented belief structure.

So let's delve into how we get the thoughts we have already ventured into and the ½ thought to work together for your benefit, [beliefs that weight loss does not exist and your language that drives new thought patterns] This is about thinking accurately and knowing definitively what it is we really want (remember no more thoughts about losing anything).

Take care of your body, it's the only place you have to live![12]

~Jim Rohn

A mental exercise to set the thought(s) in motion:

Moments after you read this, I want you to actually do this exercise even if you have to do it in separate steps.

PART I

Read this part completely first and then do it.

Sit down in a quiet place where you can begin to relax now.

Close your eyes and imagine your time-line. Your time line is your future-your present-and your past. I want you to actually see your time line up above you and out in front of you. If you see your time line going from back to front I want you to re-orient it so that it goes from left to right (where the past is to the left traveling into the future toward the right) OPTION – <u>you may want to record yourself reading this and then listen to the recording with your eyes closed</u>

This time line is simply a line that begins when you were born and flows past your existence now and into the future. And I know that for some of you when you look at the future on this line it fades and becomes fuzzy and unclear. That will only last for a few more minutes. We will clear it up as we get into completing this specific small task.

So relax, maybe even close your eyes now when you begin the exercise and see yourself floating up to your timeline and then let yourself turn to the past and notice your movement towards the past. I want you to see your life, note the events as you go back now and most importantly I want you to see yourself on the timeline – changing as you go back . . . see yourself at various stages in your life in the past. Notice the further you go back, the more ideal you can imagine your life to have been. You may not have been slender, slim or lean and you can create the image you wish in terms of what you wanted to look like now; create the ideal you.

Knowing and believing as you create this image now, that you are that person. And you may have to go back further to see clearly when that was, even now. Notice for just a second the moment in time when things began to change, especially, the transition of your body composition and your thinking. Now as you continue moving back I want you to find a moment when you were clearly that person – as lean as you will have wanted to be – slender now (I know this is relative) and stop at the moment. Place a circle around that moment to preserve and freeze it. Now reach out mentally and grab that moment-mentally and without any effort slide it over to the future side of your time line. Hold it there and note where it is because we'll come back to this frozen moment in just a second. [Stop recording if you have chosen to do so.]

Ok, why are we doing this? It is because I want you to see as you move through time that you have had many resources that helped you maintain a healthier slender body and attitude. They helped you create who you were in the past now. From the time you could understand language you have been bombarded with information, as an adult you receive over 30,000 messages a day, some of them good and helpful towards your health, you've also read, listened to and thought good health related thoughts too. As you consider what those resources are and might have been, you can begin to feel them being released from that image into your present. You can almost feel their potential stirring things inside of you now – and that's why we will come back to the image in just a moment.

Now let's quickly deal with who you created over the years (of course in your past – because you are not that person anymore). Ultimately, the strongest part of who you are and the *strongest part of your human psyche* is your identity. That is to say that what you have believed about yourself over the years is exactly what you became. Anything you have said after the words "I am . . ." is what you have and always will become. It is critical that we briefly look at what you have said and apply the thoughts you have already learned. Your identity must be altered so that your healthy, slender you can arrive and live strong into the future – right now!

If you can SEE it in your mind's eye then the probability that it can be achieved goes up tremendously

~CLE

So, who do you want to be? (Certainly if you are reading this then, fat, overweight, obese, chunky, thick, "big boned", chubby, large, huge, massive, fat behind, laughed-at, lard butt, fat, huge, big-'ol badonka-donk, BB(big boned), curvy, BMW(body made wrong), fluffy, fat man, wide load, fat and plain old BIG are not terms you ever want to associate to who you are or have anyone else do so again, ever again.)

Understand this about your brain: subconsciously, your brain knows that when you arrive into any future moment the time tense changes in an instant and becomes – NOW! In that moment *it will be* now and then that moment quickly passes and it will become a new now.

So, because that is true, then what you desire in the future will affect everything about your present. Nothing will "take care of itself" in the future. You completely control your future by what you say and who you *identify yourself* as, *RIGHT NOW!*

So, how do you want to look and feel? Again, mentally if you're reading this then, healthy, slender, fit, comfortable, mobile, physically in shape, attractive, lighter, visually appealing (to you), smaller, leaner, and confident are descriptions of how you will want to see yourself and feel.

Ok then, let's create the NEW YOU *RIGHT NOW!*

So, you already know that we always become externally what and who we identify ourselves to be internally – it is urgent and important to decide openly and cautiously, your identity. For most of us the pain of having been helplessly obese at some level in the past has caused us to ignore and deny that we might have had something to do with what we were in the past. The truth is that we were directly and solely responsible for whom we became. We were completely responsible for violating the basic laws of healthy habits, physical fitness and the laws of nature. By the way, there are always consequences for violating the laws of nature and healthiness. Think about it: If you violate the laws of gravity from 100 feet in the air then there is a consequence called gravity that kicks in and . . . well you know the rest of the story. Yes, the truth is we did it to ourselves. It wasn't depression, fear, hopelessness, the medicine, something somebody did to you, the medical condition, or your parents. And the split instant you admit it and accept responsibility, the faster your brain will allow these thoughts to actively create new neural patterns and release chemicals which make the creation of your new identity solid and lasting.

Nothing can *change* you
from the outside,
(no words, no pictures,
no person), only you can
choose to do that
and it must come
from within you.
~CLE

So who are you? What characteristics describe you? What words describe your desire, ability and willpower? What do you really look like? (Remember perception is in fact reality.) Who are you? – Healthy, slender, READY?

To help complete your identity, let's return to the moment of your time-line that we froze earlier. Once you have read this next section, close your eyes and *DO THIS* visually without distraction.) *[If you decided to record this exercise then here is where you want to pick up and begin again.]*

Go ahead and access the moment when you saw yourself as "slender", "fit" and the like. See inside of the circle you made around it. Now, I want you to access that moment and move it from the future where you placed it, over to the present; as you do, allow it to move from just a still image into a full color movie clip with borders and warm feelings and full of sounds, smells. I want you to see yourself moving about, you can hear the sounds, and feel how you feel in this moment's-image, fit and slender now.

As you allow the movie to play (and you can rewind it and play it back a thousand times in your mind if you'd like to) now, I want you to go back just a little further before this moment – and look at yourself and your life and begin to notice the many resources you had at that very moment moving forward. By resources, I mean your thoughts, your habits, your good feelings, even your take on being healthy, your motivation, incentives and even reinforcement strategies.

See, if you have already done it, been it, felt it and know that it existed then your brain knows how to access those thoughts, images, feelings, smells, and tastes so it can create what it's like to be slender again (even if you are creating it in your mind). Capture these resources now and write them down or commit them to memory. If you had any difficulty seeing, hearing and feeling these resources then answer the following question to access them. What if, you could remember now what it was like then, when you thought about being healthy, slimmer, and even knew that you had the power to control what you ate, your movements and your image of you (even if you created it)?

What would you have thought? How would you have felt? What would you have said to yourself then, if you could, remember now what that felt like to be confident and healthy minded even if you have to create it now?

Go ahead write it down if you need to ____________________,

____________________, ____________________

Recall what you see ____________________, ____________________,

____

Recall what you heard that was supportive and encouraging. ____________________, ____________________, ____________________ and remember what you thought about yourself then, right now. ____________________, ____________________.

As you access these resources that supported you in the past I want you to add them to the list of answers you came up with for the earlier question (i.e. what words describe your desire, ability, image, etc.)

Now begin to look forward into the future (on your timeline) and see yourself having all of these resources later today, tonight, and tomorrow morning. Go ahead and extend it out to the day after tomorrow and toward the end of a week. Go for it!

See yourself, THE NEW YOU NOW – Slender, Healthy, Fit, Comfortable, and Mobile, Physically in Shape, Attractive, Visually Appealing, Smaller and Confident. Do it now . . . You must do it and YOU MUST DO IT NOW.

Use the other thoughts you have learned to complete your new you! Create who you really are by sincerely seeing yourself as slender, energetic, healthy, willing and conscientious about eating healthy and moving more or as much as you can. And it's great even if you just got a sliver of a glimpse of what is possible. Do this, as many times as you have to– so that you really get this into your mind, your body, your soul and your behavior. [Stop recording]

We must use time wisely and forever realize that the time is always ripe to do the best thing.[13]

~Nelson Mandela

Once you can see yourself now, the way you were created to be – happy healthy, full of vigor, and carrying less weight – yell out, "I DID IT!" Yell out again, "I DID IT! "

CONGRATULATIONS! You have completed the ½ thought that is so critical to your success. All of this chapter has been an effort to get you to leave certain references for who you were by the wayside and know the success of it all is actually being able to truly see yourself creatively, visually, and efficiently and effectively as A NEW YOU (Your Identity)!

Just because you have done it; you have indeed begun your journey towards being slimmer and healthier. It has always been a matter of knowing that there was nothing to lose and that your thoughts and language had to be monitored and protected so that only certain thoughts and words come out of your mouth, prompting your behavior.

You are amongst an elite group of people. You are among the few people who truly realize their dreams of reducing their weight *long-term* and creating a healthier life for themselves. You can finish it and you must, to get the results you want.

Chapter Seven

Scrubbing Your Brain

Giving the Two-and-a-Half Magic Thoughts A Great Place to Live

A final task to complete your experience:

1. Find a place outside, where it would be safe to bury something.
2. Clear the area of any brush or dried debris.
3. Dig a hole 3 to 5 inches deep and about 8-9 inches round (I know some of you live in the city and this seems a little weird – but would you rather seem weird and get your results or be average and don't as well as suffer even more than you have.) Do it, if even if at a public tree mid-block in the city,[who cares!]
4. Now, take the piece of paper with your old faulty thinking and euphemisms (your repeated phrases) along with a match or a lighter . . .
5. Look at it – read it one final time aloud. Ahhhhhh!
6. *What a relief to let it out. . .*
7. NOW LIGHT IT ON FIRE!
8. Lay it in its grave along with any other secrets you might have been prompted to write down and let them BURN.

9. Once the paper has been consumed by fire – it is gone along with the thoughts you wrote.
10. Cover it neatly so you won't be able to recognize the spot a month from now / bury it and leave it there forever, Now!

You will be
who you believe
you will be-
Always!

~CLE

Chapter Eight

Breaking Free From Old Patterns

So You Can Create New Ones

So what are you waiting for, you know what to do. Go ahead and celebrate it, yell it, dance, etc., "I did it" and let the change happen as you find yourself wanting to eat healthy, eat less and energetically move more even if a little or incredibly slow at first. See, the more you live, the healthier you can become and the healthier you are, the less you'll want to eat more than you need, finding yourself eating healthier too. As well, the more you spend time thinking about your goals, and talking to yourself through beliefs, identity, thoughts, and language patterns – the faster and slender you become.

So what does it mean to be free, I mean really free from the weight and the mental slavery of being trapped into certain thinking patterns and auto-pilot behaviors.

Join me on a brief journey of . . . well, just join me.

Can you imagine life as a fish? Ok, I get it, maybe a little tough at first, but appease me for a moment.

If you could, could you imagine what life would be like living in a pond? Imagine if you will, you're a fish. A fish just like all the other fish in the pond. A pond that has murky water, and often it's so dark that you can't see very far. And of course, as a fish you are always bumping into someone because you are in such a small pond (a seemingly dark pond.)

As time goes by, and it does go by, you begin to notice that you are growing and it often appears that you have no room in the pond. You swim and swim and still, you bump into others. You decide *to swim down deeper into* the water because you know if you *sink down deeper,* there will not be as many fish to bump into as you have around you now.

And of course the fish that *swim down* are on the bottom of the pond and are always the biggest.

The thing that you learned about being on the bottom with the rest of the big fish is that the other big fish are always looking for a meal just like you were, often looking for that same easy meal, *always looking* in the past.

But it's hard (not) being among the big fish because there is really no room to grow up top and you are always on edge. Simply hanging around in the doldrums of what seems like depression and darkness. So far down that anyone else outside couldn't even know what it's like. And alone you stay, or at least that's the way it feels; so much that it feels better sometimes to stay here than to open up to the others and admit that you feel this way. "They wouldn't understand," you might think.

One day, you decide to go back up to the top of the water. You really want to get out of the murky and muddy water. But you know you have to be aware and *swim up* quickly past the other fish. You swim fast and even faster and then suddenly you get a burst of energy. *You try not* to swim that fast so you stay under control but the harder you *try not to swim fast the faster you swim.* Suddenly the water gets just a little clearer and all at once you're out of the water!

In a moment you see a whole new world. Everything is clear here. The world here has a different taste, a different smell and you hear things that I've never heard before, things that are wonderful and complete like the second thought (language/thoughts). Suddenly, just as you left the water something pulls you back into the water and you splash back down into the murky pond.

Now having experienced something incredible and hearing something that sparks your interest and remembering all the new colors and images your eyes had just seen, made you long to return to the incredible thoughts of what you have just experienced in the second completed thought. You *try not to remember the incredible experience now because you're not sure if you can reach that place again* . . . But try, *as you must* "where was this place?" You found it by accident once. Will it *be there* for you again?

You return to the deep and again you run into the same old fish. The same old stuff just keeps popping up around you. It seems like the *harder you try not to* be bothered by it, the more it keeps coming up that maybe the ones you hang around condone or accept being this way. It disturbs you to be on the bottom even when it's the top. Where you really want to be. . . . The same old dark water just seems to *keep you down.*

You wonder if you should go and see the wisest fish in the pond. The one fish you have heard about but have never seen. You've heard tales about its wisdom. Your friends tell you how dangerous it is to go near this fish, yet *you long* for help and wisdom; you want to change more than you fear.

Your journey begins just as all journeys that begin *do,* with a question. Which way do I go? You *stay there asking* that question over and over and you get nowhere because you never move from the bottom. You simply hold in place, as you swish your tail back and forth and ponder. Suddenly, it occurs to you that *you must move* somewhere and begin your search.

You swim from edge to edge. Often you stop and ask the other fish have they seen this wise fish and always they give you the same answer. "No", and now *you feel like you want* for someone to give you the answer that, "it's safer here." But you keep going and finally someone says, "What are you *looking* for?" "Well I am *looking* for answers," I say.

Perhaps if you go to the keeper of the entrance (the wise coach) of the pond, that fish will have the answer and they point you in the right direction. Suddenly it became more than a question, it is *now* an, *"I must have the answer"* feeling you're experiencing.

Once there, you notice how huge this fish really is compared to you. It's *hard not to* imagine how old and wise this fish is. I *see* scars on its sides from fish battles. It's many times your size and with such a huge mouth.

You have heard of this kind of fish, a catfish, but you never thought you would really get to meet one like this one sitting there, seemingly lying in wait.

The old catfish *opened* his eyes and suddenly you were looking at death, face to face. The old catfish says, "come closer my friend I will not hurt you". Your instincts tell you to run but your *need to know and to go beyond this place is stronger.* You move closer but not too close and you ask the catfish this question. "Well sir, where will I find clear water that tastes sweet and smells good and you can see forever?"

The catfish yawned once and says, "It's right past me and up this entrance. I will *let you pass* if you want," he said in a deep slow voice.

"But if you return I will eat you."

I ran from that catfish that day. But as hard as I *tried not* to imagine clear water, the *clear water possessed me.* It seems that the dark water is filled with gloom and has become bitter tasting, since I've had that glimpse. Finally, *I decide;* "to move is better than to stay."

I found the strength somewhere to move up again towards the edge. I could feel the sick queasy feeling in the pit of my stomach as I moved toward the entrance to the pond, where the old catfish lays in wait. I *try not* to think about the clear water, *but* the idea of *it draws me* to it.

In this life of decisions and choices, we will have the results and direct consequences of both. Freely we choose and decide and so too must we endure the consequences – good and not so good.

Decide To Be Free!

~CLE

At last my spirit possesses me and finally I swim with all of my might right past the catfish. To my amazement the old fish never moved. *It is true* what the old fish said. I could *do it if I wanted to,* finally!

Now, I am in this clear, water. It feels so good and clean, but the water is running so fast that it pulls you back toward the pond. Now you know that the old catfish is lying in wait for you. You swim harder and yet the water seems to just be pulling you back towards the pond. You look behind you and you see the water rushing past the old catfish. In your heart, fear is struck, as you see the catfish's mouth open for you, waiting for you to die. Deep within you, you search for all the strength you need to stay in this clear water and avoid the murky pond. It's there, it's always been there, that special strength you have.

Like a lightning bolt your new strength arises within you. And suddenly you're swimming upriver again.

You swim and swim and swim and you swim some more. Sometimes *you see* a HUGE rock and rest behind it for a while. You *catch your strength,* renew your spirit and you travel farther upriver to clearer water, still ahead.

Then one day out of nowhere the fast water stops. You look around you, and you *notice* how clear and still the water really is here. *How sweet it tastes* across your lips. You notice the silence, of no other fish around you, feeling the warm sun on your skin now. It's *so good to be here.* I am so glad *I listened* even when I tried not to listen to that wise old fish. I'm glad I got *out of my own mind.*

I swim around my new clear water. I *notice* how big this area of clear water really is, how strong I really am and how in this clear water I can really see how healthy I really am. In my mind's eye I see the other fish and the old life I left behind and I wish they could experience what being free of this heavy burden is really like—because *I now know.* I once carried this really huge physical and psychological burden and no one knew what it was like, what it tastes like, what it smells like, and how good it feels to have the sun shine clearly on my healthy face.

So much room here, so few fish *you think,* if they only could *move;* BE FREE!

Your past does not dictate your present. However, your future can and always defines your past. The moment to choose what you will have is now.

~CLE

It is better to experience several moments of discomfort and or pain (make changes, even if uncomfortable) than to suffer years of living mediocre.

~CLE

If you are going to have to go through painful moments in life to get what you ultimately want, you might as well get a wanted result or reward for it.

~CLE

By the way, you will know how well you are living by how healthy you are and the level to which you are achieving your dreams, targets and goals.

~CLE

Chapter Nine

How Bad Do You Want It?

Everything Costs Something – Are You Willing to Pay

I've had the honor of professionally coaching since I was just out of college. The privilege of coaching athletes, politicians, business owners, medical and health care personnel as well as regular people like "you and me" and seeing them get the results they want is an incredible pleasure and rewarding experience. I've also seen many people who said they wanted a certain result and never even got close to that result. They either did not have the drive, the passion or the heart to persevere (all have the capability to persevere but not all cultivate the ability to do so). They would start and often never finish the effort, to get done that which would have led to the results.

So I want to know before you actually launch into this chapter: do you have what it takes? Are you committed? Can you finish? Do you really want it? Are you willing to go all out? Will you finish? Are you willing to push through what stops you? (OR) For what has stopped you in the past, do you know what it is, and will you push through it in your present and future?

HOW BAD DO YOU WANT IT?

We all have desires and wants; we all have things that we think about and jokingly say we want to achieve. And some of us talk about those things all the time. But, how committed are we? How badly do we really want it to happen? Does it burn inside of us like cold breathe in the winter? Does it mean more than anything in your world at this moment? How badly do you want it? When you wake up, is it what you are thinking about, when you go to sleep and or nap is it one of the things you're thinking about?

How badly do you really want it?

Whatever you imagine is your reality, thus whatever you can achieve.

~CLE

I was in a conversation recently at the local hospital where I worked, with a colleague whom I have come to admire. The gist of the conversation or at least the element I found to be insightful was related to the idea of "how badly do you want it." Here's part of that conversation—

Kelly: I want to be healthy but it's so hard.

Christopher: Concrete is hard, metal like that paperclip in your hand is hard. Human thoughts are pliable, changeable, and not necessarily hard.

Kelly: I know that makes sense but I just can't seem to get it going again.

Christopher: Ok, so what does that mean?

> Kelly: Well, even my doctor says I've done well, and I need to just get the next twenty pounds off. I just need to get going, I'm stuck and don't know how to start.
>
> Christopher: Here's a thought, you've already taken off twenty pounds, which is rather significant. So, it's not that you don't know what to do or how to do it, it seems like it's an issue related to how badly you want to. Something stirred you the last time, and what's true is that it's not showing up at the moment. If you can figure out your motivation and discern how bad you really want this, you can take off the next 20 plus pounds easily.

At this point a physician walked by and overheard enough of the conversation to politely enter the conversation and contribute the following thought:

> Dr.: "Interesting thought, I get it – I used to be obese. (Both of us express shock and she continues.) You know when I was twenty six years old I was seriously obese, I was almost 100 pounds more than I weigh now. And I was showering one morning when it occurred to me that I could no longer live like this; I was embarrassed and hopeless until that moment, and even afraid of whether I could actually get rid of the weight. But, this was that moment – when everything had to change. I couldn't be fat anymore." ("I took off almost 77 pounds over the next year)". And I spent the last 26 years obsessed (NOTICE HER WORD CHOICE, "obsessed") with keeping it off"

Confronting your past allows you to freely move into your future now!

~CLE

Here is a doctor who is at least 52 years of age based on her comment and REALLY, gets what it means to want something so bad that she describes it as an obsession. Although, I had seen this woman from afar in our work when she spoke these words I knew and recognized the kindred spirit. She knew what it meant to want something in a way that causes you to ache, dream, burn with passion, and be consumed by thoughts that translate into congruent, consistent action. Her description was the perfect demonstration of the answer to the question "how bad do you really want it?"

It is unfortunate however, that most people never get to feel that level of passion for something; where nothing else matters at that moment-mentally, socially, physically and maybe even emotionally. I knew that regardless of our backgrounds, our responsibilities, and stressors we could crack a smile with each other knowing that we have traveled the same road to get to the point of obsession, and change.

She went on to say:

> Dr.: "When you are obsessed with something it doesn't mean that you don't have a life, it just means that you're willing to pay the price to keep or to obtain whatever it is you're passionate about. For instance, I went out of town this past weekend and struggled with whether to eat certain things. In the end I chose to let my hair down and indulge myself in different kinds

> of food and other things I would not have normally eaten. Yesterday morning, even though I didn't feel like it, I went to the 'Y', and worked out. While I was working out, I thought about the weekend, and how much fun I had, realizing that my work out was simply the price I was paying for an incredible weekend. Other times I realize that I can't be like everybody I call friend and can't even do what they do. I have to be unique to achieve what I want – their dreams are not mine and they will never understand my passion and my drive . . . very few people really get what this means in life."

Naturally, I was amazed to hear this philosophy because I absolutely get it. The idea that often "to be massively successful at something, you may often have to travel alone and not be fearful of doing so." This was refreshing that someone understood the uncomfortable place of what it means to really go after something. Noticing that she understood what it feels like when you have to do it by yourself, for yourself and literally leave even your closest friends behind . . . (sometimes temporarily and sometimes permanently) was remarkable.

So the notion of how bad you really want something is not just a colloquial term, or hypothetical question. It is a question designed to gauge whether or not what a person says they want is congruent with what they're willing to do to achieve it, and whether or not they're willing to pay the price for the victory in having their dreams come true.

The difference between a successful person and others is not a lack of strength, not a lack of knowledge, but rather a matter of will.[14]

~Vince Lombardi

Often this means learning to enjoy life (sometimes) alone without dependence or codependence on another person for a while. It could mean that we're willing to learn about ourselves long enough to be good at being ourselves rather than being absorbed into someone else's personality, absorbed into someone else's drama and even living out the life they plan for or advise for us. Certainly when we find ourselves working diligently on their life issues and not our own passions, then we have lost temporary hope of achieving our own dreams. Another way to look at the matter is, that many people use a person's weight as a way of keeping them under a certain kind of control so as to benefit themselves. It's here, in my opinion, where dreams can be won or lost. Ultimately, you have to decide that being the new you is worth everything to you. It's in this defining moment that many people go outside the boundaries of success and into the fields of distractions.

Ultimately, everyone is motivated by something. Many of us however, are not aware of what it is that actually motivates us. What motivates you as it relates to your passions or the things that are important to the quality of your life, are often unknown? In any case, however, motivation is the key to why we do nearly everything.

It is the fuel that provides the reason, energy, willingness, and follow through to achieving nearly everything we set out to achieve. So this notion, of, "How bad do you want it," has to be a way of life, a quest for a place you're not at or have been. If you have been there, and are consciously aware of it, you would know what it's like and will want the experience of it again. What does it take to answer the question, however, so that you get the result you want? I believe there are three things you must have and understand to want something bad enough, that it is all you think about, all you are focused on, and all you live your life for, within a given time frame. According to most performance coaches these three parts are necessary, critical and vital.

Firstly, you must have the courage to change, and often stand alone. Some people describe this as heart; some people describe this as "guts" or intestinal fortitude, and ultimately it is the want to that drives all of us to do anything and everything. Do you have that courage? Are you obsessed? Are you willing to fight through the challenges and tough times to get the result you want? Are you ready to do what it takes, even if this means sacrificing your time, energy, friends and even your resources to get the results that you want? What if it costs you physical effort; what if it costs you diligence; what if it costs you sleep; what if it costs you social gatherings, events and relationships? Do you have the strength, the guts to fight through this to achieve your results, because it's going to take real heart and lots of guts to do so?

Many people say that the secret to completing any task is beginning. I tend to differ . . . It matters not that you began a task, or a goal, or dream. It does matter that you finish it and get to enjoy the rewards of having done it!

~CLE

Secondly, as Eric Thomas says, "you must be able to sacrifice at any moment what you are for who you can become." It is the notion that no matter what's happened to you, no matter the state that you find yourself in and, no matter how difficult it is to get to the place where you feel healthier, look healthier and ultimately are healthier you have to want it like nothing else at that moment. As well, your past "never", in no way, equals your future and so between the present moment and your future, which will occur at any given moment past this one, you must be willing to give up who you are, to have who you want to be.

Even in the moments of depression, frustration, confusion, and seemingly a state of inability or loneliness you have to find a way to push through these moments. So this too requires a commitment that in some ways can be very tough for most and requires the intestinal fortitude to overcome the natural unwillingness to give up ourselves to become someone else. Ironically, in this instance as we deal with taking off weight; when we have that end result we will in fact have become someone else.

Thirdly, the idea of "how bad do you want it", because it's related to change always has a measure of pain associated with it. This pain is in most instances temporary; it could last for a minute, an hour, a day, or even a year. Eventually, it will dwindle, as something else is most likely going to replace it.

A. If you quit, you will have to live with never knowing if the next moment of your effort was that moment when things would change for you.
B. If you quit, the pain turned regret might last forever
C. If A and B, (knowing the next moment could be it and having no regrets) are in place and if you are prepared, when the pain subsides you'll be able to replace it with what you've prepared, to go in its place.
D. When it seems like you cannot take it any more that's when you're on the verge of breakthrough. So, hold on.

Pain by the way can be the greatest leverage for change in human behavior. We do not change easily most often. However, extreme logic and pain are two of the greatest motivators toward change in the human personality.

At the end of pain by the way, is results and success if you hold on and persevere.

So, how bad do you want it, requires you to have laser focus. Your behavior has to be very intentional and deliberate. Your maturing thoughts must support you with an understanding that all humans are created equally and that some work more diligently at becoming, doing, and finishing the work that is their (your) passion.

So, HOW BAD DO <u>YOU</u> WANT IT?

When you want it as much as you breathe, then you will be successful.

Many of us say that we want to change the way we feel, change the way that we look, change our eating habits, take off excess weight, be able to run again, feel better about ourselves, change our wardrobe, do some things we haven't been able to do, change our health status, get back to certain weights we've known in the past, become who we believe we are capable of becoming, achieve a certain life goal and or simply be a healthier version of ourselves; not everyone will.

In spite of what we might say, and what we want, many of us are not willing to do what it takes to get this done. We've been unwilling to get up an hour early or carve out some time to exercise so that we ultimately, have no reasons to use the excuses "it's too hot, it's too cold, I'm tired, I don't have a gym membership or access to a gym" and ultimately get it done. Or, many of us are unwilling to go to bed an hour later, so that we can go walking in the evening. We've refused to go to the gym, we've turned down the invitations from others to work out and instead we sat watching TV, lying around, eating unhealthily, and feeling sorry for ourselves.

There are some things in life that you simply have to do once, you decide to do them.

There is NO QUESTIONING

There are NO HESITATIONS!

~CLE

When you want something as bad as you want to breathe, then it becomes very easy to sacrifice a few minutes of sleep, a few minutes of time, a few social appointments, sitting around on Facebook, Instagram, Pinterest, twitter, tumbler, google +, and OMG, the other 290 social media platforms that could occupy all of our time. You'd be willing to DO SOMETHING about your health or other goals in life.

When you answer the question "how bad do you want it?" the desire to change and become your potential has to be a burning desire inside of your belly that emanates to every other part of you. Every limb, every digit, every brain cell, every neuron, and every hair follicle has to *be on board. To change* that which has not been easy to change (or you wouldn't be reading this book, and you would've already changed it), you must be consumed with the idea night and day. All humans are motivated by something, every single time we do anything. Ultimately everything we do is designed with some purpose even if just to be silly. It is what makes us human.

I know all of the above to be true because, after gaining 75 pounds of mostly fat during my experiment, I struggled with nearly all of it. I was told, I looked fit . . . I was told when I would have conversations at the start of my reversal that I didn't need to change anything, that I was fine and that all I needed to do was stay muscularly toned. Ten (10) waist sizes ago, I knew the truth deep inside. It was a constant battle to want the change and be free from the physical pains, the mental discontentment, the lack of motivation and even the distress of high blood pressure, knee pain, headaches, and even the embarrassment of not being my best. I didn't want it bad enough and the more I read the manuscript for this book the more I realized that not wanting it bad enough was the key factor for my lacking effort. Suffice it to say that when my "want it bad enough, was high enough nothing in the world could stop me . . . nothing.

The plan to do it came with ease, the resources that were already there surfaced, and just so you know, I didn't even go to the gym for six months, which I was paying for monthly. (All of it happened right at home except for one week, when I went to the local high school and ran sprints and walked on their track)

Furthermore, our ability to purposefully or intentionally change who we are by virtue of our personality, our physical being, and our habits makes us unique and fully human. This goes without saying that you and I can in fact have in most cases whatever we want as long as we are willing to do what it takes to get that very thing.

Sometimes it requires us to learn; sometimes it requires us to experience pain for a short period of time; sometimes it requires us to sacrifice sleep; sometimes it means that we have to work on our plan instead of going to the beach, to the pool, golfing, out to eat, or having a drink with friends. More than less, it may mean that we have to move when we'd rather sit still; it may mean that we have to eat less of the thing that is our favorite and exists in abundance.

This is the beginning of what it means to want it more than you breathe, and even then the question still lurks as a reminder that until you achieve your goal completely, you will have to answer it, if only to yourself:

Today I noticed a penny on the ground.

I remembered my karate instructor (Eric Blaize), trying to teach me to be more aware of everything around me and to be in proper form; he used to say, "Keep your head up! Where you are looking is where you will go. Your vision sets your destiny!"

What are you looking at? Keep your head up, find your destiny, and *stare at it until you achieve it.*

How Bad Do You Want It?

As I think about what it means when someone asks "how bad do you want it?" I'm reminded of a story told by my good friend Eric Thomas.

He shared the story of a young man who says to a wealthy guru, "I want to be on the same level that you're on, I want to have as much money as you do. I want to have the same access to any and everybody. I want to do the kinds of things you do."

In a welcoming but solemn tone the guru said, "If you want to be on the same level as me then meet me at the beach at 4:30 AM tomorrow morning."

Thinking that this would be a great business meeting, the young man showed up at the beach at 4:15 AM, in his suit and tie, thinking that he would beat the guru there.

As he walked out onto the beach he noticed that the guru was already there waiting. As the young man approached, the guru asked "so, you want to be on the same level as I am?" "I do", said the young man. "Then walk out into the water with me," said the guru.

The young man dressed in a business suit, took off his shoes and uncomfortably began to walk out into the water. As he walked out so that the water was around his knees. He turned to the guru who said to him, "please continue walking with me," as he moved deeper into the water.

As the water rose around the young man's waist, he began to think "this man's crazy, all I wanted from him was to show me how to make money, I just wanted to know what he knew, this is crazy." As the guru moved even deeper into the water, the young man found himself in water around his shoulders.

With no conversation being held the young man began to look at the guru wondering why in the world he was being asked to follow him into the deeper waters. Now, with the water around the young man's neck rising up to his chin, he looked at the guru who was much closer to him than before, and just as he looked, the guru reached over grabbing his head, and pushed him under the water.

The guru then held him there under the water as the young man flailed and fought to get free, trying to resurface. It seemed like an eternity . . . (and) . . . just before the young man was about to pass out, the guru let him up from beneath the water. As the young man gasped for air fighting the water that was flowing into his mouth and nose, the guru turned to him and asked, "What did you want more than anything while you were under that water just now?"

Gasping, the young man replied, ". . . to breathe, I just wanted to breathe."

The guru calmly asked him, "Did anything else matter in that moment?"

The young man, still gasping responded, "No, nothing else mattered, I just wanted to get some air. I only wanted to breathe."

The guru slowly turned and began making his way back to the shore with the young man close behind. Just as they had gotten back to where the water was around their knees the guru turned to the young man and said, "When you want it as bad as you want to breathe, then you will be successful."

WHAT IS IT THAT YOU WANT?

If you just want to be happy—lower your expectations. If you really want to be happy, raise them. If you want the happiest life possible, simply expect greatness!

~CLE

Chapter Ten

So What Do You Do Now? Finish!

There is a cost to living a mediocre life. It's typically not one that will bankrupt your finances (although it could); it's not one that is going to cause you public scorn or shame (although it might); it's typically not one that will cost you family and friends (although it could lead to that); and, it is not one that will cause you concern, distress or dissatisfaction, although it very well should.

There are many people who cruise through life enjoying it, without being responsible for much or even taking responsibility for very little. They never actually make a difference in the lives of others or even think about what it means to really live in the moment. Ultimately, when it's all said and done, we all are driven by our individual psychological needs that must be met in order to achieve any behavior. It is ultimately, our behaviors or lack thereof that leads us to deterioration, mediocrity, self-actualization or a really fulfilled life.

So, what does this mean? Well, a big part of living is at some point being or becoming aware that life has a terminal point and how we live in between our beginning and end matters. It matters that each of us indeed has a purpose. Ultimately, to achieve a purpose we must be able to live at a functional level such that we recognize (even if not fully defined) that there is some greater purpose to living.

At this level we engage with life and those connected to it. As well, *without your health,* your psyche and all of your brain functions will become focused on keeping you alive, and helping you maintain homeostasis (the balance of life).

What am I saying? You may not, others may not and in general anyone may not expend any energy on being healthy. You may not, others may not, and in general anyone may not spend any energy on being healthy, (stated 2x to make sure you got it . . .) However, the human brain in and of itself is designed to keep you alive. So, it makes sense that at some "higher level", we all have a purpose, and at a basic level, our brains being designed to keep us alive, both together, suggest that it makes sense to go ahead and be healthy on you travel on life's journey so you can *live your purpose well.*

With that being said, and it's obvious that I am pushing you to contemplate and or become more health aware (conscious); I want to acknowledge that I am aware that I have not spoken about several things related to the idea of being healthy.

1. I have not addressed specific caloric intake, work-outs, eating plans, metabolism, and or in depth opinions on surgeries and procedures. (there will be a tad bit towards the end of this chapter)
2. I have not walked through the specific psychological needs that humans have and how they prompt us toward the aforementioned habits and results.
3. The things we TOLERATE we will never change in our lives; which is to say that if you only desire a change at a superficial level and you are not prepared to *be the best you can possibly be* then you simply won't be and you will have superficial results.

   (No tolerance for bad results.)

4. When your reasons overpower your desire to WIN in whatever you're doing, your desire becomes the leaking tire on an old car due to be towed to the junk yard. (No one cares, and the excuses eventually become part of your being crushed.)
5. The *opinions of others* are just that – their opinion. You don't own them and have no obligation to adhere, abide or perform according to them.
6. Lastly, YOUR PAST DOES NOT EQUAL YOUR FUTURE, it never has and it never will.

So that you know, all of these specific things get addressed in the Ultimate Weight Loss blog, coaching plan and seminar. As well, it will be covered in the Health Mastery coaching series. In the meantime the upshot of what is intended here is that you are in charge of what happens with you. Regardless of what is happening to you (Perspective, Perspective, Perspective,) you are responsible for your opinion and your perspective.

So, once you have the ideas in your head that allow you to change your life, your health life can change now. At the least you will be standing in a clearing where you can more easily create who and what you want to be or do. The motivation to do what needs to be done is often what is lacking and the way in which you take advantage of being propelled towards the life you want is often what's missing.

In many cases, Tolerance, Motivation and a lack of clarity about where you are going, influence the process of achieving. And from this place of lack of clarity, we often ignore information, don't understand true decision making and fail to set solid directions for our movement.

Over the next few moments I will be as Transparent, Forward and Direct with you so that you get to observe in you a new way to really create the most incredible life you could possibly have. Your work will be to employ the lessons learned and live it out with the vigor and intention you were created with.

So, how do you live with healthy intentions and intense meaning?

Our bodies are constantly changing in an effort to find healthy & optimal functions. Why not support your body in its amazing capacity & hard work![14]

~FLK

<u>Here's A Philosophy to Consider:</u>

Live like a S.T.A.R.

S– Show self-control and discipline in eating and exercising

T – Take Responsibility for your life and your health

A – Act Safely and decisively – know what you are after

R – Respect Yourself and Others to the MAX (take it easy on yourself when you don't meet your goals and encourage yourself on the way to achieving them) – know that others typically do the best they can with the resources that they have, so be forgiving when they fall short of your expectations or encouragement. This will be a great stress reducer related to your weight reduction efforts.

1. MOVE: DO SOMETHING Walk to the mailbox twice; walk around the house or up the stairs five times today; sit

still and move your arms; with your legs move them 10 times apiece. Gain your health back by being determined – for each exercise add one more repetition or movement each day.

2. FIND YOUR PURPOSE simply put, find your purpose and you will have found all of the motivation you will ever need to *change* now!
3. LIVE . . . I mean fully LIVE. I've worked in fields where death showed its face more than I ever cared to see it, as often as I did. You are alive – choose to create a lifestyle of responsibility to do something about every condition you experience, so that your days alive may be extended to their fullest capacity.

It is in the moment when we think beyond the anxiety, <u>the fear</u> – the very thing that stops us – (that in most cases <u>is not</u> even <u>real</u>), that we excel and LIVE LIFE TO ITS FULLEST!

~CLE

When you are challenged, or you find that you are not getting the results you want or you seem to be thinking repetitive thoughts that are unhelpful, use the following technique from my friend Joseph McClendon (Life Coach) to stop the behavior. With this technique you can redirect the behavior and then reinforce the behavior that you want.

The S.T.O.P. Technique

S – Say the words STOP! -to yourself when you need to get the thoughts and or the actions to desist from occurring. (Say it forcefully like you really mean it.)

T – Take a deep breathe, or Take a moment to move yourself from the physical position you are in; change it.

O – State the other behavior you actually want to be doing or thinking instead of what you actually found yourself doing.

P – Pat yourself on the back for catching yourself.

REINFORCE the behavior you want to have happen. (i.e. "great job Christopher, way to catch yourself and stop these thoughts")

Ultimately, once your goal is set, pointing you in the direction you want to be going in, begin moving in that direction

Remember, in your doing so – live! The bottom line, stop living as if you're not going to die – that's right, STOP LIVING AS IF YOU ARE NOT GOING TO DIE
Because you are – You ARE!

SO LIVE NOW!

CLARITY
Get it – Keep it!

~CLE

You were created to be healthy. Your job and role as a human is to BE.

~CLE

The Accountability Partner: Why You Might Need a Coach

The annals of time reminds us that to be accountable to someone is one of the best formulas for being successful.

Throughout history have you ever noticed that every great athlete from the beginning of time has had a coach or training partner that helped them achieve greatness and or championship status…? A Chinese proverb reminds us that "To get the best results from people it is better to light a fire within them than to light one beneath them," (which suggests that even in the oldest of cultures the value of someone coaching and or keeping you accountable is important and recognized as highly valuable.)

The truth is that you might be able to achieve all of your health targets alone and by yourself. Some people can and most don't. After-all if it were true that it was easy to do by yourself we would have an epidemic of healthy people versus the obesity epidemic. We would have slight to a few pounds over our natural-weight populations versus what we currently see.

So can a coach really help you achieve your results? Why do you even need a coach or accountability partner in the first place? What can a coach really do for you? What can they do for you that you can't do for your-self? Do you really need an accountability partner or a coach? What is the real value of a coach?

If you do not have a coach why not?

You have to ask yourself are your health targets and goals worth trying and trying to achieve and not getting the results you want or would it be better to simply have a person you are accountable to and someone who is going to hold you to whatever you commit to, to help you get what you want. A coach's job and or an accountability partner's job is to take no excuses and push you to be your best (period) regardless of your excuses and reasons why you can't.

I will never accept less than the absolute best from any of my coaching clients or partners. It is my goal to help them understand that they were created not just to be good at something but to be great at it– this includes their health. -Christopher Eaddy, PhD, NLP

Perhaps the following will allow you to understand why in the future, now, you should and will have wanted to have a coach to help you get your best results. I do not advocate for you a coach because I am one, (and am a good one at that), I advocate for a coach because even though I have coached nearly 1000 people in the last five years, I too have a coach-

So what can a coach really help you with;

- A really good coach can help you <u>determine what is truly important</u> in your life and then help you stay focused on the important what, where, when, and how's related to those important tenets
- A Coach will help you identify where you are, where you want to be and what is creating the gap in between
- A really good coach creates space for you to be able to clearly see your true self and to be able to see your incredible capabilities.
- A good coach helps you set health and fitness targets, so that you have ongoing achievement milestones to step onto and successes to build upon
- The best coaches finds **your motivation** and **compels you** to desire achieving **your goals**.
- A coach drives you towards your best, purposeful thoughts, actions and keeps you committed to what it means to be your healthiest you

- A good coach helps you develop your belief system, so that you can believe that you are not only good in your efforts to achieve healthiness but that you can be great at it
- A coach or accountability partner can guide you to build a structure of accountability, So <u>You Will Reach Your Goals</u> and then what you've learned will support you so that are ensured to sustain your commitment

Yes my coaching clients say I'm tough on them and hold them to an incredibly high standard for themselves- and they will also say they are successful at achieving their goal's dreams and milestones. -Christopher Eaddy, PhD, NLP

I have had the pleasure of coaching top level CEOs, CIO and even professional athletes. They are at the top of their selected professions. Yet, they, are wise enough to know that to stay at that level and to want to be better at what they do, they need someone to push them and remind them that they are capable of more. As a means of being your best; why wouldn't you want someone to push you;, to remind you of what motivates you; to question you and prompt you to achieve, grow, and excel, even when you're tired and simply don't want to be your best

Interestingly, there are studies upon studies about coaching, that shows, those who have a life coach and even organizations that have them have a higher financial IQ and income impact than those that don't – apparently that's why CEOs, VPs, and other leaders to include Doctors and political leaders have strategists and performance coaches; (seemingly they are smart for their effort)

Have you ever thought about why most people never achieve greatness?

Well it might just be that it's not in their everyday – nearly every moment thoughts. As a coach it is my job to remind people of their capability to be great as an everyday thought. Being great is an attitude, a desire, strong enough that it forces you to prioritize decisions and choices that get you results. Unfortunately many of us settle for okay and maybe even good. Life is short and great is within reach for all of us. Often times a simple nudge from an accountability partner or a coach makes a difference between average, good and living a really great life.

When looking for a coach, ask questions and listen closely for what you don't want to hear and for you don't want to see if you are meeting face to face. In many cases when you feel like the person is rough around the edges and would clash with your personality – that could be the very coach you need… They should be able to articulate their methodology and the frequency of contacts with you which should diminish over time because their mark of success is that you do not need them anymore.

Your coach should help you:

1. Gain clarity on what you really want, how you plan to achieve it and milestones you will achieve along the way
2. We all have things we don't know, even coaches too. The scotoma or blind spots are only made visible by those who are trained to generally know what they are, and know how to listen and identify them. Coaches can help you find the blind spots that keep you from experiencing expedited success. Coaches help you figure out what you don't know, and they clue you in to things you may not be able to see. They will be honest with you because they are only vested in your success not the goal itself
3. Maintain course when it gets tough. Sometimes we all get sidetracked and lose our way in terms of strictly staying the course. As well, it does not help when we are moving and active and we're not moving forward.
4. Develop- A good coach helps you become better at being you. Ultimately, you'll waste less time – engage in activities that are more meaningful and enjoy the work of being an achiever.

5. Be fierce in obtaining your health goals. The truth is everyone has something they want to achieve. Some get there much faster than others. Why not you? Where you are is not where you have to be so….
6. Gain skills that you can use for the rest of your life in other situations. A good coach helps you deal with life's situations with solutions that easily apply to life's general situations making it easier to keep moving when things get tough long after your coach is gone.
7. Be your best and learn to be happy in all of the situations you might find yourself in. This includes the struggles that come when you are trying to achieve your health goals and targets. Considering my journey from 236 to 310 pounds and then back down to 229, I know the struggles will come and they are real to have and have to be dealt with. You will have better results with a happy disposition, when you will have had someone with you on the journey.

So, why don't you have a coach? In the shortest admonition and strongest suggestive tone I can give you… you should hire a personal trainer or a coach to help you get to your results so you get there faster and you have accountability in guaranteeing you get there.

How much would that be worth to you?

My personal interview with Joe Greenwood, World Renown Personal Trainer

I talked with Joe Greenwood after he had just started a morning boot camp program in his hometown near Pittsburgh, Pennsylvania.

I knew he had immense experience in helping others get the health results they were seeking. I asked him several questions about his methodology and how he had gained so much success. I recorded many of his answers so that I could share them with you here. The following is part of that conversation.

1) **What is the easiest exercise I can do (assuming the person is really obese with poor wind conditioning and mostly immobile) to help reduce my weight?**

   Joe: Being obese, a person with poor wind conditioning, mostly immobile or a person with a disability makes exercise challenging, but not impossible. You should see your doctor or health-care professional before you choose an option that might be suitable for you to engage in. Together you can decide whether you might be able to do some home exercises or if using a pool would be the best option for you.

   Ultimately, if you will choose to be active and you do have some kind of a serious limitation there is a device (called an arm-ergo meter or arm cycle) that many physical therapists use for exercising patients with low mobility or limitations. This is very useful for people who can't stand and you can still get a cardio workout using only your arms. It's a great way to get an aerobic exercise without having to stand.

   Here are some other suggestions of exercises for people who have limited mobility. Remember to consult with your health provider before starting these or any workout routine.

   1) Roller chair workout (great for people who can't walk or stand)

   . Find an open area without carpet
   . Use a chair with wheels on the bottom
   . Propel yourself using your legs around the open area.
   . Start at 1 minute and build your endurance.

a) Pilate rings

. Put rings around your wrist and try to make them spin in circles.
. Sit on a stability ball and make figure eights with your hips and spin Pilate rings with your arms.

* Turn on some music while exercising to "amp" up your pace and to make it a bit more fun.

Pool workouts are also great. Water is one of the best fitness tools around. It provides resistance which strengthens muscles and boost cardio intensity. It also supports some of your weight, making workouts easier on your joints. The pool is a great fat burner. You can burn a higher level of calories in a shorter amount of time in the pool. Just walking in the pool is a great workout because of the resistance.

2) **Questions 2 & 3 combined: Why is it important to use legs as part of exercise especially if I want to reduce my weight?**

If you're not doing leg exercises for "weight loss" or overall muscle gain you are at a slight disadvantage when it comes to taking off the unwanted weight. Because leg muscles are responsible for so much movement, they can burn a lot of calories- fast, and they are among the most important exercises to take off the extra weight. Energizing leg muscles with the right exercises will help you quickly shed the pounds, as well as tone your legs and lift and tighten your Gluteus Maximus (your butt muscles or glutes). The best exercises are multi joint exercises, meaning that your hips and knees are moving.

The main muscle that moves these joints are the glutes, hamstrings and quadriceps (front and back of the thighs). The best exercises are squats, deadlifts, and lunges and any of their variations. Single joint exercises such as leg extensions, leg curls and calf raises target individual muscle groups and they can be beneficial depending on your goals. As far as taking off weight is concerned you can use multi joint exercises like squats, deadlifts and lunges to work all of the leg muscles at the same time which will save you time. (Simple squats done 'til you can't do any more and then deepening them and increasing them in to sets over time are an easy way to start these multi-joint exercises.)

4) Do I have to use weights in my effort to reduce my weight?

In order to reduce weight it's important to increase your rate of metabolism. Lifting weights increases your body's rate of metabolism and keeps it raised long after the activity is completed. This is because your body has an increased demand for oxygen as a result of the workout and thus registers an increase in the metabolic rate. Muscles are an important factor in raising your metabolism. A pound of muscle can burn up to 20 calories a day whereas a pound of fat can only burn 5 calories a day. Since weight lifting helps build muscles and also burns fat it has a dual benefit in reducing weight. In addition weight lifting workouts also help strengthen the bones and increase endurance levels. You get optimum results when weight lifting workouts are combined with cardiovascular activities.

5) How often should I exercise?

The answer to this question depends on your fitness level and what your target or goals are. If you are a beginner and new to exercise it is advisable to follow each exercise day with a rest day to allow your body to repair. If you're used to exercise and wish to exercise on consecutive days try alternating between different forms of exercise; for example weights on Monday, cardio on Tuesday. I would suggest working out at least 4 days a week.

Put a day of complete rest or cardio in between each weight training workout. Of course, interval training, cardio sessions and a proper meal plan all have effects on the results you get. We do have to remember not to go overboard and over-train. It's about balance and rest which is just as important to your results as working out or exercising.

The following is adapted with permission from an article written in the Soul Pitt Quarterly Print Magazine, in Pittsburgh. *(www.thesoulpitt.com, 2/24/2016)*

"Most of us start the New Year with some sort of resolution, however, as time passes those resolutions go right out the window. Johnstown native Joe Greenwood is here to remind us that one particular resolution is a must and should absolutely be carried on throughout the year. That vital resolution is the goal for a healthier lifestyle.

Greenwood believes that health is wealth and he has made it his mission to help people not only get into shape, but stay in shape as well.

"There's nothing more important than your health. We put so many things above ourselves sometimes, but at the end of the day you can't really enjoy those things if you 're not healthy," said Greenwood.

Coaches like Joe are available to guide you even if you are far from Pittsburgh, He like others can use virtual means (computer, cell phone, etc.) to reach out to you and help you get the results you want.

Joe can be reached at by going to the youwillseeresults.com website on the resource page.

Chapter Eleven

Nutrition

You Are What You Eat

I had, early on, believed that I would not write much about nutrition when I first completed this book. My background is in psychology, law enforcement and minimally medical. I have learned to be incredibly good at the craft of profiling, personality diagnosis, analysis, and even teaching. My work has been focused on giving people mastery over their thinking and circumstances. My work has been bringing people back from the brink or providing comfort, motivation and inspiration.

The first part of this book achieves just that. It is the effort to have the habits of unhealthy thinking brought to a place where a person's new thought processes revolutionizes their health. It achieves its results by offering a different result for those reading and hearing this information. In almost an incredible twist of fate, understanding what it means to be fit and healthy physiologically, it became increasingly urgent and important that I speak about health and fitness together.

Additionally, I have been unable to let go of my thoughts on nutrition even if they might have been superficial compared to the literature out there. In thinking about nutrition, my philosophy was rather simple at first; your body either seeks to assimilate what you put in it to help with further functioning of the body; or it seeks to eliminate what it doesn't need. The next level of thinking about nutrition has to be the considerations of what really happens when you put certain items into your body either expecting certain things to happen and in some cases expecting certain things not to happen. Of course, if you are consuming food and other supposedly nutritional products all with the intention of managing your health, your weight and your well-being, then as purposeful as your intention has to be, your understanding of your potential outcomes has to be. So enough philosophizing, let's get to the facts of nutrition.

Ultimately, when thinking about nutrition there are several things of which we must have a good understanding in order to appreciate, change, and utilize its power. First, let's define nutrition. According to the 12th edition of Nutrition, by Sizer and Whitney, Nutrition is the study of the nutrients in foods and in the body; sometimes also the study of human behaviors related to food. The absolute importance of nutrition is to gain an understanding that nutrients interact with the human body adding a little, or subtracting a little, day by day, and thus changing the very foundations upon which the health of the body is built.

When fear becomes your friend and never again something that stops you it can be a long-term motivator

~CLE

Furthermore, knowing what nutrients are in our food and what roles they play in the body is key. That leads to managing meals and understanding how to evaluate nutrient content in packaged and marketplace foods.

Of course if you are growing your own food, you will want to know how to balance what you're eating to be able to sustain your healthiness. This effort is also important in managing illnesses, if it can be managed with eating styles. You will also want to reasonably avoid heavy usage of foods that do not offer valuable support for your health and fitness goals.

So, let's begin by talking about what it really means to achieve this state of weight reduction which would essentially be eliminating stored fat and creating lower amounts of you over time (as it relates to nutrition.)

You are what you eat? Well, maybe. And, if that's not the case then there can be no doubt that what you eat will grossly impact who you become, how you get where you are going health-wise, as well as how you live once you do get to "who you'll become." After all, we all have a need for food (sustenance) in order to survive.

First we have to deal with some myths, and urban legends to get to the truth of what you need to consider when it comes to food.

I swore to myself I wouldn't write about nutrition and even exercise. However, some things can't be left alone and must be talked about or mentioned at the least. So, let's look at what you most likely were taught to think about some foods. For instance, many of us have been told to eat "healthy whole grains," we were advised that they were better than white flour products. Well, let me let you in on a dirty little secret of agribusiness: This is a myth and simply not true. Yes grains might be better in general yet because the wheat and grain of yester year are no longer what we eat today there are some risks that most of us haven't known about. It's not the same grains. It is not the wheat of our grandmothers' day because it was changed.

As we already discussed, wheat and grains were changed in the 1960s and 1970s by agricultural scientists. They hybridized various strains thousands of times. They mated wheat with other grasses (wheat is a grass).

Your life is going to be lived whether you are a active or a passive part of it.
~CLE

They subjected wheat seeds and embryos to the process of *mutagenesis:* the use of chemicals, gamma rays and x-rays to induce mutations. These methods pre-dated the methods of genetic modification (gmo), and were crude, imprecise, unpredictable and, in many cases, worse than genetic modification.

Many varieties of wheat that we eat come from plants that are no longer tall, but are short and stocky and high-yielding. Changes in outward appearance were accompanied by internal genetic and biochemical changes. One crucial change is the forms of the protein, gliadin. Gliadin, when digested in the human gastrointestinal tract, is degraded to small peptides that can bind to the opiate receptors of the brain – yes: *opiate* receptors, not unlike morphine or Oxycontin.

Gliadin-derived peptides, however, don't make us high, nor do they provide pain relief; instead they may only stimulate appetite and *cause us to eat more.*

Do you remember this tid-bit from years ago: "According to a nationwide survey: More doctors smoke Camels than any other cigarette"? In the mid – and latter 20th century, there was a national discussion about the pleasures and health benefits of smoking, to studies documenting the damage to health caused by smoking, to executives denying any wrongdoing to Congress, to uncovering concealed documents demonstrating the industry's knowledge of the adverse health effects of smoking *decades* earlier.

I believe we are reliving the tobacco experience with wheat in its place. I think that smart food scientists stumbled on the potential *appetite-stimulating effect* of the gliadin protein in wheat more than *25 years ago.* How else do we explain why wheat can be found in so many processed foods, from tomato soup to licorice? In 1960, you would have found wheat in bread, rolls and cake – obvious places that make sense. Go up and down the food aisles in your local supermarket in the 21st century and you will find that huge numbers of canned, packaged, and frozen foods contain wheat in some form: licorice, taco seasoning, frozen dinners, beef jerky, cereals, and even salad dressings – you'll be hard pressed to find processed foods that do *not* contain wheat. Is wheat that necessary for taste or for texture? I don't know. I do think it's there for a specific reason: to stimulate your appetite and increase sales.

By the way it's in the baby aisle, the detergent and cleaning item aisle, the meat aisle, etc.

I think that by putting wheat in nearly everything, the food industry ensured that you come back for more. Just as tobacco manufacturers increased nicotine content of cigarettes to help ensure addiction, so adding wheat to processed foods might help create an addiction to all things wheat. Not only could that add up to a lot of calories and a lot more food consumed, it could add up to a lot more weight. Alongside these changes in wheat, we have observed a nationwide increase in weight. An explosive surge in diabetes has followed the rise in obesity.

We are now in the midst of the worst epidemic of diabetes ever experienced by humans, and rates are continuing to climb, threatening our children and grandchildren's health.

I believe that the gliadin protein of wheat ensures that wheat products, such as whole grain or white breads, bagels and muffins, are *addictive:*

They generate a need for more . . . and more, and more. Gliadin may act like an opiate with its own form of euphoria and its very own withdrawal syndrome when you remove wheat from the diet.

In my opinion, the inadvertent transformation of wheat gliadin into a potential potent appetite-stimulant, recognized quickly by observant food scientists, brought us here, to this overweight, diabetic situation. It is a situation that now plagues Americans and much of the rest of the developed world, all while we are advised to eat more of these GMO grains.

A true sign of being intelligent is not how you think, but how you think about what you imagine.

~CLE

FACT:

- Wheat is considered one of the most hardy and high yielding foods for the food industry
- Present day wheat is resistant to: heat, a lack of water (drought conditions), most insects and all because of chemical modifications
- Interestingly, wheat is not considered genetically modified although it is hybridized (you decide)
- More interestingly, is that most grazing animals won't actually eat current day wheat as it grows in the field, to include: birds, cows, wild turkeys, deer, wild hogs, goat, and other grain and seed eating creatures . . . so you decide whether it's a product you want to eat a lot of, if at all.

Like current day wheat, many foods are filled with things most of us don't know about. Here's a few tips that will help you manage better the foods you eat; first thing's first:

Avoid buying the foods that reside on the store shelves at the level of your eyes down to your stomach. – These foods have the highest manufacturer profit margin – the store's highest profit margin foods and usually the products are made from the cheapest ingredients and with some of the products, the worst ingredients. Let's examine a few:

Fat-free – Where fat is removed from your food products, typically something has to replace it or it wouldn't be cost efficient to give you more of the actual product and not charge you more. So, what is it that replaces the fat in fat-free? Normally, it's sugar or sodium that replaces fat. Understand however, that there is such a thing as good fat. It is necessary for energy, hormone development, your hair, and remember those fat soluble vitamins like A, D, E, and K. Normally the sugar content is worse in these foods than actually eating pure fat. Which leads to the issue of fat itself; *saturated fat is the problem not fat in general as a food.*

Saturated fat exists in many natural forms like the fat on your pork chop or the fat on your prime rib and in these cases they're not all bad. On the other hand any fat that turns to a solid at room temperature, like lard can obviously be bad for you (imagine it in your stomach, intestines and or permeating your linings and into your blood stream and then turning solid.) Unsaturated fats like the ones you find in some oils, avocados, and some nuts are in fact good for you. So the *issue is not necessarily fat. It really is sugar and or sodium.* Let's see if we can simplify the issue with sugar.

When you consume more sugar then you will use ("burn" calories is usually the term we use to describe calorie usage because of the heat generated in movement or exercise to actually consume or dissipate a calorie) *it gets stored as fat calories.*

NOTE TO REMEMBER: when there's extra sugar in the blood – the pancreas sends out additional insulin to get that sugar out of the bloodstream. It either converts it to energy or stores it as fat for later use. This is typically how sugar leads to weight gain because your body is forcing your system to store more calories as fat calories when you've consumed too much sugar.

Here's the bigger problem – sugar spikes in your blood system – and your blood system responds by producing more insulin – this tends to handle the blood spike really quickly. When your blood sugar spike is handled really quickly then you tend to have a sugar crash. When you have a sugar crash your energy level diminishes and you feel sleepy and sluggish. When you feel sluggish and sleepy from the sugar crash – your body releases neurotransmitters that suggest that you need nourishment – this is largely based upon the amount of glucose/sugar in your blood system. When the neurotransmitter called neuropeptide Y (NPY) along with Grelin which circulates in your blood, interact – the desire for sweets and starchy food goes up – when Grelin rises, your appetite rises too.

So just imagine that you're sleeping and your glycogen stores and blood sugar stores get used up. This causes your brain to release NPY, so that when you wake up NPY and Grelin have interacted and you typically desire breakfast. If you miss it, an intense hunger arises, maybe even a binge kind of hunger.

This leads us to the issue of the no carb diet. This diet typically does not work because it really prompts the overeating of proteins and in many cases the overeating of fats which can be obtained through high-fat meats, fried foods, and even some processed foods. Most of the foods related to a high protein diet are high calorie value proteins. Calories are calories however, no matter how you look at them – eat more than you burn and it gets stored. When it gets stored it's typically stored as fat.

Now let's take a look at artificial sweeteners in our foods that are designed to be helping our weight control efforts.

Fact:

Aspartame the most popular sweetener in "diet foods", worsens your insulin sensitivity and that may not be the worst of the facts shared in the next few moments about aspartame. (Understand that these are facts with references for you to further read about, yourself, not just my own inflection of thoughts). I'll come back to the insulin impact in a moment, but first, these facts help you better decide what you want to put in to your body as you work to be healthy.

Firstly, Aspartame is often billed as a no calorie sweetener. It does have calories: 4 per gram

Secondly, Aspartame is made from the waste products of E-coli bacteria. After the benzene alcohols are added and water is infused, derivatives of methane are added and then some of the benzene alcohols are removed . . . talk about genetic manipulation

Thirdly, Aspartame turns into formaldehyde [in your body and the last time I checked, in simple – "that's not good"]. (I wanted to say more here but after reading at least 15 articles as far back as 1905 on formaldehyde, I thought it would be best for you to read at least one so you would see it's not my opinion but a formal document from a Food and Drug Administration hearing) It's scary and you might be shocked, and, you'll definitely get to decide for yourself.

http://www.fda.gov/ohrms/DOCKETS/dailys/03/Jan03/012203/02P-0317_emc-000196.txt

In summary, Aspartame rapidly stimulates insulin and leptin involved hormones with satiety – over time too much leptin causes your body to lose sensitivity to it and the body does not hear the message to stop eating, burn fat, and may include sensitivity to the flavor of sweet on your tongue.

Ultimately you can develop leptin resistance – which increases your visceral fat, hunger, fat storage, and carries an increased risk of heart disease, diabetes, and metabolic syndrome – What is metabolic syndrome you ask: Abdominal obesity, Elevated blood pressure, Elevated fasting plasma glucose, High serum triglycerides, Low high density cholesterol (HDL), Diabetes, Cardiovascular issues to include Cardiovascular disease and Heart disease

Even in mid, 2017, a report came out from the Canadian Journal of Medicine suggesting that artificial sweeteners when used consistently were linked to weight gain, heart disease, and other health related issues to include: diabetes, high blood pressure and heart disease.

Rice: I like rice and grew up eating a lot of it as a family staple. I'll be short and to the point here. Be choosy if you decide to consume it. Know that what you want is rice as pure as you can get it and be sure that it is not GMO (Golden Rice) because it will cause you to accumulate weight if eaten over time and simply may not be safe. You decide.

Dr. Mehmet Cengiz Oz (Dr. Oz) weighs in on some of the myths related to things we've learned and heard over our lives.

You were created to Wake up,
Kick butt, and;
Repeat

FACT: Eating Fat Makes You Fat

The name says it all: Fat makes you fat, right? Wrong! Eating a small amount of fat actually helps you feel fuller faster as it triggers satiety (or fullness) signals, causing you to eat less overall. Not just that, eating the right fats aids in the absorption of healthy vitamins. Seek out the polyunsaturated fats you'll find in liquid oils, like canola and safflower oil.

Unlike saturated fats, polyunsaturated fats won't raise bad blood cholesterol levels and may even reduce the risk of a heart attack. To get your healthy fat fix, also look for omega-3 oils from fish, krill, seafood, algae, flaxseeds and/or walnuts, and olive oil, which is a source of both monounsaturated fats and omega-3s. The fact is of matter is that it is the kinds of fat you eat not fat itself that makes you fat and is the problem in weight gain.

FACT: You Burn Fat Faster by Exercising on an Empty Stomach

Starving yourself before you exercise isn't only ineffective, it may be harmful. In a recent report a study concluded that your body burns roughly the same amount of fat regardless of whether you eat before a workout or not. However, you're likely to lose strength-building muscles by exercising on an empty stomach. Not only that, without food to fuel your workout, exercise intensity and overall calorie burn are reduced.

On the other hand, when you exercise with some food in your stomach, you're burning fat instead of muscle, leaving you with more energy and a higher calorie burn. Be sure to eat 30 minutes before exercise, preferably a liquid-like yogurt or a protein shake so your body can make nutrients readily available for your workout. If not your body may think you're trying to starve it and cause it to go into save the fat mode.

When the body recognizes useable food in the stomach and uses it, it will then satisfactorily begin burning fat for the additional energy needed rather than muscle mass (protein).

FACT: Gender Doesn't Matter: When it comes to weight reduction. Men may appear to lose weight faster than women at first, over the long run however, things balance out. Men tend to have more muscle mass and undergo fewer hormonal changes, which allows for an easier burn-off of those first few pounds.

Research shows, however, that, over time, weight reduction evens out between the sexes so long as you stick to a healthy diet and exercise routine. Remember, healthy results don't matter over a week or even a month – they really add up and matter over the years.

If you only had one of something and actually used it daily and you needed it to function in life, would you care for it?

(...a thought and note of question from Your Body!)

FACT: All Calories Are Created Equally

A calorie is a calorie but does not automatically equal a calorie when it comes to quality. Some calories are more filling, leaving you feeling full faster so your appetite is gone in a flash. Other calories are less filling, keeping your appetite going and going and going.

You want to seek out the first type of calories, so be sure to replace the less-filling saturated fats that you'll find in butter and fatty meats with the more filling, polyunsaturated fats found in sources like avocados and nuts. You'll get the rich, delicious flavors you crave without packing on unwanted pounds.

However, when it comes to unused calories and the way they get stored . . . a calorie is a calorie.

In thinking about being healthy, taking off weight and nutrition, at some point we have to talk about bloating.

If you've got bloating so bad you think you might just pop, put an end to it now, that's right, today. Many people wake up with flat bellies, only to find that by the end of the day their stomachs are distended and painful. Fortunately, gastroenterologist Dr. Robynne Chutkan who works at a digestive center in Maryland shares her plan to eliminate hidden causes of tummy trouble and help to get rid of the bloat.

Step 1: Start your day with an anti-bloat elixir She says, "many people are jinxing themselves right off the bat by reaching for bagels or sugary cereals first thing in the morning. These foods clog up your system and set you up for day-long gas buildup. Instead, get your system moving right away by blending together this fiber-rich elixir (www.doctoroz.com/videos/anti-bloat-elixir) that helps food move through your digestive tract.

Aim to get 25 grams or more of fiber a day, but if you normally eat a low-fiber diet, start slow and gradually increase the amount. If you notice a little extra bloating at first, don't be deterred – most people's bodies will adjust to increased amounts of fiber over time."

Step 2: Supersize your lunch

Her second step suggests that "many people eat their biggest meal at dinner, (guilty as charged, and working on that however), but eating too late at night can cause a log jam in your gut. To help beat bloat, you should enjoy a three-course lunch instead. Make sure your lunch includes about 10 grams of fiber to help keep your food moving.

Here's a good example of a fiber-rich, delicious lunch option:

- First course: Salad (add in all your favorite veggies and a light dressing)
- Main course: Grilled fish with sweet potato and a cup of steamed broccoli
- Dessert: A cup of fiber-rich fruits like raspberries and/or blackberries o Important to note, eat the fruit first . . .

One nutritionist has suggested the following: Eat like a king at breakfast; eat like a queen at lunch and like a younger prince at dinner- their logic is that if you eat more food at breakfast (full of fiber), you will feel fuller longer and be more active, burning more calories throughout the day and less into the evening as you'll be eating less too.

CONSTIPATION AS IT RELATES TO BLOATING

Typically, other than severe medical conditions (namely, fecal impaction), most people eating three meals a day and being properly hydrated, eliminate waste from their body every two days if not once a day. Of course this is often dependent on what they are eating and the fact that metabolism and internal body mechanics slow as you age. If you find yourself constipated and feeling bloated then perhaps you might consider the following ideas to get things moving – pun intended.

- Adults need to do at least 60-75 minutes of aerobic activity at a minimum every week. This type of exercise stimulates the contraction (peristalsis) of the intestinal muscles, which is extremely important for effective waste elimination.
- Eating plenty of fiber to keep yourself regular can also help. If you suffer from constipation, eat more beans, berries, flax

seeds, prunes, celery, cabbage, peppers, close to raw broccoli, etc. Fiber in general makes your stool retain water, so it will definitely be much softer and heavier thus more apt to pass from the colon.

- A trick I learned from a nurse colleague during treatment of a patient suffering from a month's worth of impaction – (imagine not being able to go to the bathroom, #2 for a whole month . . . (thanks Ricky)) – is using a simple stepping stool under your feet when eliminating. Sitting upright on the toilet can cause constipation in and of itself, simply because of the recto-anal angle posture.

  Simply put there is a curve at the end of everyone's rectum, a 90-degree angle that easily stops you from pooping yourself just because you have the urge to eliminate. However, that angle only slightly straightens when you sit on the toilet. That leaves many of us "straining" to eliminate our colons. Adding a stool to your bathroom ritual makes for a better pooping posture for eliminating and just might eliminate some of the constipation.

  Ultimately, with a potty stool, the weight of the torso presses against the thighs and naturally compresses the colon. The gentle pressure from the diaphragm aids the force of gravity and voila! The puborectalis – (The fibers that form a sling for the rectum) relax, allowing the rectal angle to straighten out and the bowels to empty completely. Whew, I'm actually glad to get that subject straight.

- Not sure I'll have to use this remedy, but having researched the topic – I found this food consistently in the literature. Parsley – This herb that tends to grace our plates as a visual, and in both forms parsley "juice" and "fresh" parsley have been found to be an effective remedy for constipation. Perhaps, based on the studies at the American University in

> Beirut where researchers found that parsley does in fact have laxative qualities we may have a healthy, natural remedy.

Lastly, if you're an acupuncture, acupressure homeopathic practitioner there is the Cv6 method. Although, I cannot say I was a believer at first and I am regular by the way, I opted to try what I am about to explain and within thirty minutes was in the bathroom (porta-potty to be exact.)

The ancient art of acupressure suggests that the Conception vessel 6, as it is called, is essential to know about because it allows the bladder to release, the colon to release and stimulates some kind of energy force similar to adrenaline being released, all increasing our vitality. As it relates to poop however, here's what you need to know to try and employ this technique.

Step #1 – Make sure you're near a bathroom (thank God for the porta potty)

Step #2 – Just measure three finger widths below your belly button. Then take your first three fingers and press the Cv6 acupressure point as you take deep breaths.

Step #3 – Continue pressing until you feel the need to go. Be patient as it can take as long as 3 minutes but as little as 10 seconds other times!

HOW TO GET YOUR FAT TO EAT ITSELF . . .
(Metaphorically speaking)

If you've got stubborn fat that's been living with you a lot longer than some of your close family, here are some thoughts to help you get it moving. By choosing the right foods, you can prompt your fat into a self-burning furnace once you train your body to metabolize it well.

Monounsaturated fatty acids, or MUFAs, are found in some of the nature's most indulgent foods, including nuts like cashews, almonds and pecans, nut butters, avocado, olives, olive oil, coconut oil, and even dark chocolate. Oddly enough, a study from the American Diabetic Association found that consuming a diet rich in MUFAs over time decreased some belly fat (remember that belly fat can be a precursor indicator of healthiness).

These MUFAs can help improve insulin sensitivity, which will help control blood sugar control and help avoid and even help treat diabetes.

To make these monounsaturated fatty acids beneficial for you – eat them as a part of most of your meals and try as much as you can to get close to half the required fat calories you need daily from the MUFAs.

Here's some good portions and foods to use as a rule of thumb:

- 2 tablespoons nut butter
- 2 tablespoons olive oil
- ¼ avocado
- 10 olives
- 2 tablespoons nuts
- A quarter cup of dark chocolate chips

**As is with all humans;
What we focus on
grows because we tend
to move towards it,
what we focus on
becomes real and what
we focus on we get
more of –
Monitor What
You Focus On!**

As a wrap up on the topic of Nutrition I want to return briefly, to the issue of wheat. I realize I was rather critical of wheat and it comes from reading, reading, reading and experimenting. So, instead of offering my potentially skewed opinion, I have adapted some of the answers to popular questions about wheat from someone who has studied it extensively as it relates to healthiness. (Cardiologist, Dr. William Davis, MD)

Q: I thought whole grains were good for health? Is that not true?

A: A simple fallacy in logic led to this incorrect conclusion.

The epidemiologic studies that were used to argue that "whole grains" are good for health did nothing of the kind. What they showed was that, when processed white flour products were replaced by whole grains, there was an apparent improvement: less weight gain, less colon cancer, less heart disease and less diabetes.

Turn off the poor me, sorrow – not good enough, I failed channel, nobody loves me channel and turn on- The I'm good at something channel – Right now!

#Livefully

> This is an example of replacing something bad – white flour products – with something less bad – GMO whole grains – resulting in an apparent health benefit.

Studies suggest that replacing white flour with whole grains may contribute to minor reductions in weight and conditions like colon cancer, heart disease and diabetes, but it does not necessarily follow that whole grains are better than no grains.

What should have been asked in the next logical progression is: What are the effects of no grains? We have to look elsewhere for those answers.

- The notion that whole grains are good for health is therefore based on a simple blunder in logic. While grains, especially wheat, do indeed provide inexpensive calories on a large scale for the world's diet, their consumption invites compromises in health if they are in the modified versions and consumed in large amounts.

Q: Why would someone lose weight by removing wheat from the diet? Isn't it just a matter of losing the calories from wheat products?

A: No, and in fact I encourage consumption of high-calorie foods such as fats and oils.

- The weight loss effects of wheat elimination derive from the loss of the gliadin protein of wheat. According to the results of several studies already mentioned in this book, from the 1970s and 1980s, gliadin is degraded to small peptides then bind to receptors in the brain. The effects can vary from individual to individual, with effects that include mind "fog," triggering impulsive behavior, and anxiety, but most people experience appetite stimulation, causing an increase in calorie intake.
- Wheat also contains a unique carbohydrate, amylopectin, a largely responsible for the high glycemic index of wheat containing products, whole grains included. Blood sugar highs are followed by precipitous blood sugar lows, a pattern that develops over an approximate two-hour cycle. Blood sugar lows are accompanied by increased appetite. This means that people experience a two-hour cycle of satiety and hunger throughout their day, having to eat to respond to the blood sugar low.

By the way, this is the basis of what Dr. Davis – a cardiologist's work was based on. He was looking at patterns of what his diabetic patients were eating when they experienced blood sugar spike (glycemic index increases), Bread / wheat was the most common factor he found in asking his thousands of patients to self-report.

- Lastly, there is another protein in wheat, wheat germ agglutinin that may block the leptin receptor, one of the hormones of satiety, in effect turning off the normal controls over appetite (Wow!)
- Lose the gliadin-derived opiate effect, the two-hour cycle of hunger, and the leptin blocking effect, and appetite plummets back to a natural level designed to provide sustenance, not indulgence.

Perhaps the wheat and grains controversy is still unclear and we may never know how accurate the studies are. One thing for sure, If we balance our indulgence with it, we will be better served in the long run.

Your ATTITUDE determines your perspective. Your PERSPECTIVE will determine your reality and we behave according to our REALITY – (#Attitude)

~CLE

Chapter Twelve

Eating Clean

Ensuring Your Results

As mentioned several times throughout this writing, the idea of eating clean food can only be beneficial for you; good for your skin, your organs, the function of your organs, and your overall health. This EATING PLAN ALLOWS you to eat all the "natural" foods you want. This way of eating is also the best way to reduce your weight if exercising is difficult or challenging to do.

As often as you can eat cleanly, your body will learn to burn the sugars, and convert the fat stored in your body as energy sources. The excitement is that this type of eating promotes fat storage burn, which ultimately reduces your weight. Here's a list that might help you move toward eating a bit cleaner.

CLEAN EATING - SHOPPING LIST

- Artichokes
- Apples
- Artichoke hearts
- Asparagus
- Bamboo shoots
- Bean sprouts
- Broccoli
- Brussels sprouts
- Cauliflower
- Celery
- CousCous (Israeli)
- Cucumber
- Daikon
- Eggplant
- Leeks
- Lentils
- Lychee
- Beans (green, kidney, garbanzo)
- Greens (Collard, kale, mustard, turnip)
- Rice protein powder
- Mushrooms
- Green Tea
- Okra
- Onions
- Peas and Pea pods
- Peppers
- Radishes
- Rutabaga
- Squash
- Sugar snap peas
- Swiss chard
- Tomato
- Water chestnuts
- Watercress
- Zucchini
- Cabbage (green, bok choy, Chinese)
- Salad greens (chicory, endive, escarole, iceberg lettuce, romaine, spinach, arugula, radicchio, watercress)
- Ground flaxseeds
- Brown rice
- Olive oil
- Balsamic vinegar (or other preferred vinegar) for salad dressing

A Few More Things to Consider / adapted from Prevention Magazine, [February (2016 p. 60)]

As you can see from the list if you are going to eat clean, you have to start off with a few items, either from growing or shopping that are, single ingredient foods. From nearly every piece of data it appears that the healthiest foods in simple, have one single ingredient. You're encouraged to get: fresh produce, whole (non-GMO) grains are better if you can find them and they're within your budget, nuts, legumes, plain natural yogurt, eggs (free-range if you can find it), fish and meat.

**Those who do,
find a way
to
Get it done. Those
who don't, find an
excuse to explain
the lack of results.
(Choose to do)**

Another consideration is that *sugar is the enemy* of healthy weight reduction – especially, when it comes to eating clean. Added sugars can be known by other names than just "sugar". I do however, without overwhelming you, think you will be surprised by some of the names as well as the number of them. I also think you will recognize some of them . . . and begin to notice more of them in your food's ingredients lists – here we go:

Data from DHHSS (U.S. Dept. of Health and Human Services) and the Food Label Movement:

Fructose	lactose	Fructose sweetener
maltose	malt syrup	high-fructose corn syrup
Honey	liquid fructose	fruit juice concentrates
cane crystals	brown sugar	Anhydrous dextrose
Cane sugar	corn sweetener	corn syrup

Corn syrup solids	crystal dextrose	evaporated cane juice
Maple syrup	malts	mannitol
Nectars	pentose	raisin syrup
Ribose rice syrup	pancake syrup	rice malt molasses
Raw sugar	sugar syrup	white sugar
Carbitol	corn sweetener	concentrated fruit juice
Diglycerides	disaccharides	evaporated cane juice
Erythritol	Florida crystals	fructooligosaccharides
Galactose	glucitol	glucoamine
Hexitol	inversol	isomalt
Maltodextrin	malted barley	rice syrup solids
Sorbitol	sorghum	sucanat
Sucanet	xylitol	zylose

Whew, are you tired yet? This list doesn't even include all of them – there's way over a hundred of them . . .

SUPERFRUITS and SUPER-FOODS are mostly hype, nearly 100% of the time. First let's be logical and practical. If there was a super food and or a super fruit wouldn't every overweight person wanting to take-off weight in the world be eating it right now. Secondly, wouldn't some company or companies be involved in making sure there was enough of it to make them wealthy?

Be OK Cooking At Home. I have been amazed over the last several years at the number of people I have met who eat out at least four to five times a week. How else can you control your portions (in restaurants – bigger is better)? How can you control what additives go into your food? Unfortunately, we are used to eating everything on our plates and not wasting any of what we pay for. As well, we don't know all of the additives that are being placed in your food perhaps other than the usual culprits which you can ask to have absent from preparation (artificial fruit syrups on desserts, artificial sweeteners in the low calorie foods, reused oil from vats – used to sauté and cook other foods, artificial coloring and flavors [they have to be able to make money – real ingredients cost real money], refined sugars/ corn syrups, etc.).

Never in your life
will you be more
successful
than the moments
when you know
what and how
to do something
and then simply
– choose to *Do*
It.

EATING STYLES AND COOKING TYPES

CLEAN EATING

Registered Dietician, Jaclyn London from Good Housekeeping, in an article from March of this year, offers some thoughts to clarify what clean eating is and what it recently has been interpreted to mean. "What it truly meant when the phrase eating clean was introduced as a style of eating was that the food categories consist of mainly whole, real foods.

This includes vegetables, fruit, grains, plant-based protein, animal based proteins-(direct source versus processed or pre-packaged/ cooked meats), nuts, seeds, and oils. A further implication of the term "clean eating" is that the foods should be as close to its natural state as possible, versus factory manipulated."

The idea of clean eating normally implies that the food should be cooked at home when cooked at all. The idea continues that clean eating means you are continuously aware of "what is in your food."

You do your homework and know where it came from by checking your sources, you read the labels and have a general sense about how your food generally gets to you. According to London, a major concern for all of us is that, "sometimes the idea of clean eating has frustrated her because it implies that anything other than "clean eating", means that all else being eaten is unclean, or non-hygienic."

Furthermore she explains, that if "your product is labeled healthy and clean but is 90% full of a trendy version of oil or sugar, it's still not providing a healthful, educated choice regardless of whether it is labeled clean." She gives the example of, Agave, which she says, "is no better for you than any other version of sugar." Coconut oil, she says, "is still a mostly saturated fat (even when used over kale salad as an example); cold-pressed juice is still a concentrated source of sugar (and not very nutritious); and that vegan chocolate pudding is still dessert – not breakfast and does include lots of sugar", she adds.

If you are going to attempt to eat cleaner she recommends the following tips:

1. VEGETABLES

"When you can figure out how to make eating more veggies work for you, then obsessing about "clean vs. dirty," becomes irrelevant. Just find a way that works for you and your family to eat more veggies, and then just do it. It doesn't mean "eat veggies only" or "all the time." It means make more of your meals veggie-based."

2. EMBRACE THE IDEA OF TRANSPARENT vs. CLEAN

She says that, "if you are to eat something like candy although it is not by any means congruent with the hashtag #cleaneating, it clearly is what it says it is." (I Like Her Next Comment) – "No one bought a candy bar *thinking* it was anything other than a treat!) Is your candy bar a candy bar, or is it *pretending to be an energy bar.* If it's the latter, put it back and go for the real thing" she says. Let candy be just that when it supposed to be, candy.

3. EAT FOOD FOR FOOD'S SAKE AND NOT THE CLAIMS (it makes)

Food brands create a lot of their wealth by putting "health" claims on their products – some of which are totally legitimate, while others are ridiculous. (Why are "eggs" suddenly "gluten-free"?) – They've *always been* gluten free and unless they are GMO'd at some point they *will always be* gluten free.

4. STOP THINKING ALL PACKAGED GOODS ARE A NEGATIVE

London suggests that, "a lot of experts have pushed this term as a catch all for meaning bad – Not always true", as she explains. "There are some important exceptions to the idea of packaged foods with short ingredient lists or pronounceable items being bad for you. A great example is 100% whole-grain bread that is stuffed with tons of 100% whole-grains and that has a component list that can barely fit on the package.

However, things like the quinoa and amaranth (two of-the-more ancient grains) are downright unpronounceable for some." As well, (I tend to eat) canned fish as a single ingredient with water, but there's also cooked-dried beans or peas in a to go package, as well as *pure* squeeze peanut butter out of a packet, or even a hardboiled egg on a stick in a package," which are not all necessarily bad for you."

Perhaps Moms and Dads were on to something when they tried to get us to eat our vegetables, just maybe…

CARB-PROTEIN BALANCE

In a HEALTHY EATING (healthyeating.sfgate.com/) article entitled,

How to Balance Proteins and Carbohydrates by Registered Dietician Erin Coleman, in the San Francisco Chronicle – the case for the protein – carbohydrate balance offers the following:

"When it comes to immediate fuel for the human body we cannot live without carbohydrates. It is our main source of energy." As mentioned earlier in the book too many carbohydrates – to include sugars and refined foods and we'll end up over-weight and even obese. Proteins on the other hand, are essential for building muscle, energy, growth and development and the body's ability to heal. "The trick is balancing it so that we are not on a fad or "diet" craze that is more injurious than helpful." Avoid high protein low carbohydrate eating plans and of course avoid low protein high carbohydrate eating plans too.

Erin refers to the Institute of Medicine's recommendation of "45 to 65 percent of your daily calories from carbohydrates, and at least 130 grams of carbs every day. She states the following as an example; "if you eat 1,600 calories per day, 720 to 1040 of those calories should be from carbohydrates, which equals 180 to 260 grams of carbs per day. If you eat 2,000 calories per day, you need about 225 to 325 grams of carbs each day."

From the same source she quotes that, "our protein requirements are at least 46 grams of protein each day for women, men should consume at least 56 grams and that pregnant and nursing women should eat at least 71 grams of protein. Based on these recommendations, you should consume 46 to 140 grams of protein when consuming a 1,600-calorie diet and 50 to 175 grams of protein when following a 2,000-calorie diet for optimum health.

Sometimes, when you find out that foods are not the way you thought they were – it should make you vow to never be hoodwinked again

From a study and article from a 2007 study published in the *Journal of the American Medical Association,* comes, what I believe, may have been the catalyst for the high protein-no carb based eating plans that swept the globe in the early 2000's.

This report concluded that "increasing protein intake and limiting carbohydrate consumption can help overweight individuals reduce calories to achieve successful weight loss." A 2012 study published in the "British Journal of Nutrition" found that women who consumed a reduced-calorie diet showed better improvements in weight loss, body fat, lean body mass and chronic disease risk when they consumed a diet with a 1:2 protein-to-carbohydrate ratio.

An example of this ratio is eating 75 grams of protein with 150 grams of carbs when consuming a 1,200 calorie weight-loss diet, or consuming 100 grams of protein with 200 grams of carbs when following a 1,600-calorie weight-loss plan." Again, for optimum health THERE MUST BE A BALANCE as the imbalance will create issues over time.

Good sources of dietary protein include lean meats, fish, seafood, poultry, eggs, cottage cheese, reduced-fat cheese, seitan (for non-celiac allergy eaters), tofu, nuts and seeds.

Examples of healthy, high-carb foods include non-GMO grains, fruits, corn, peas and potatoes. Nutrient-rich foods high in both protein and carbohydrates are low-fat milk, soy milk, yogurt, legumes and some nuts.

A TRUE MYSTERY

REDUCED FAT, LOW FAT, FAT FREE and LIGHT VERSIONS

Eating foods where you monitor the fat content should in fact be something all of us do to remain healthy. However, it can be confusing and often times deceiving when trying to navigate food labels, claims and what's good for you and what is not.

I will try to simplify this issue in as short a writing as possible.

According to the FDA (Food and Drug Administration) labels that boast these claims must meet the following criteria:

- "Low-fat" foods must have 3 grams of fat or less per serving.
- "Reduced-fat" foods must have at least 25% less fat than regular versions of those foods.
- "Fat-free" foods must have less than 0.5 gram of fat per serving.
- "Light" foods must have either 1/3 fewer calories or 50% less fat.

Hopefully that is a tad helpful and I understand if it leaves you more confused or at least unsure (I was all three when I first read these.) Instead of having to occupy your time and energy on the details of memorizing these percentages and amounts, perhaps you can allow yourself to be contented by understanding that we should focus on eating and consuming "good fats" versus detrimental ones.

For instance "fat-free" can and does in most cases leave food with a taste not preferred by most of us.

Food manufacturers know this and in the place of the missing fat, place other ingredients in the food. These ingredients include sugar (most often), salt, flour, MSG (monosodium gluconate – [a thickener and flavor enhancer]), and salt which in most cases increases our caloric intake.

Here's one of the greatest examples from my research that will floor you when it comes to the idea of a no-fat solution in foods. I sincerely do not intend to gross you out if you have consumed it. However, in the production of a particular style of milk which I will name at the end of this paragraph there is little to no fat.

1. It was initially a waste product for the industry.
2. When discovered that it could be marketed as a no fat product, it became something designed to make money versus being an incredibly healthy product.
3. Its natural color is actually grey and is thickened and colored by a derivative that is placed in it under high pressure, which oxidizes cholesterol and is known to cause plaque build-up in human arteries. To the known nutrition buff, oxidized cholesterol is an antioxidant. However, under pressure, this form is denaturized (proteins are destroyed) so badly that the body doesn't even recognize it and it causes inflammation (FDA does not require it to be listed in the ingredients.)

4. According to the book GMO DECEPTION by Sheldon Krimsky and Jeremy Gruber (2014, Skyhorse), because of the way feeding occurs for milk producing animals, sickness prompts the use of antibiotics but pus and blood are allowed up to a percentage of parts per millions by the FDA in this product
5. There are GMOs (Genetically Modified Organisms) designed to cause higher yields of this product (a growth hormone developed from itself – rBGH).
6. It has almost ZERO nutritional value

- It will not help you reduce your weight. (It was, before being discovered as a marketable product, fed to pigs to help them increase their weight before slaughter.) READY? Wanna know what it is?

Skim Milk

So, to ease the pain and confusion of dealing with fats in food (in general) refer back to the section on FAT and be clear in understanding that obviously we do not want to consume too much of it and that we need it to be healthy. The key is to be informed and balanced in our intake and avoidance of it.

Never accept that ignorance is bliss because it can also be deadly…

~CLE

Chapter Thirteen

Understanding Food Preparation

The Good, The Bad and The Ugly

HIGH FIBER

Fiber is recommended as a regular part of our nutritive eating plan. However, if not balanced can be detrimental. In simple, fiber is not absorbable in our gut. Additionally, it is not digestible. What that means is that there is little nutritional value in fiber itself. On the other hand fiber helps us to create bulk to prompt "poop", clean the colorectal areas of our internal food pathway and to (at times) supplement our food with a natural filler allowing us to experience satiety or fullness.

In the end it helps us refrain from eating high calorie foods on a regular basis, so it does have a valuable place in our eating plans – just not as a staple to be eaten all of the time. The key is to make sure there is a balance in the amounts we consume so we are getting the proper nutrition we need to maintain healthy weights and to have healthy systems.

BAKING

There are some inherent advantages to this cooking style. Namely, there is a lower fat content in foods that are baked because of the heat process. Also, flavor can be enhanced in foods that are baked versus boiled, or steamed. Because of the time it takes to cook baked food one should be careful not to overcook the food as it will dry out and be void of flavor. In this instance if time is critical, as in the food was prepared for a particular time and then ends up being "ruined," a quick fix to obtain a meal may lead to a not so healthy option.

Many times it's not what we eat, but, how what we eat has been prepared.

(a candy bar is not so bad occasionally – deep fried in butter with a two inch breaded crust sprinkled with confectionary sugar – not so much...)

FRYING

Frying is often convenient and even low cost. From a healthy perspective it is a low fat absorption option related to cooking and an eating style. There seems to be conflicting evidence supporting both perspectives of good and bad when it comes to frying as a cooking style.

I mean clearly studies show that people who fried their food over a ten year period (40,000 people) were shown to have *no greater* risks of heart disease or premature death than those that didn't and insulin levels in obese women were found to be positively affected from frying foods. One bit of information collected but not taken in to account until after the studies were done, was what kind of oil was used to fry the foods. Olive oil and Safflower oils are the clear choice based on the results of other studies, but, the type of oil or fat is just one factor that can affect the healthfulness of a fried food.

Other possibilities include how it's fried (deep or pan), whether the oil is reused (the less, the better), and how much salt is added. The only part of the study that wasn't accounted for was the overall eating style of the participants which may have had some impact on their healthiness overall. In the end frying foods was not seen as a negative in the studies, especially when the frying was done in a pan versus deep frying.

STEAMED

In general, steaming your food has always been a preferred choice in food preparation particularly because it preserves the protein in the foods-(especially vegetables). As well, most of the taste of the food, namely vegetables is preserved. One of the issues with most cooking types is the vitamins and mineral are cooked out of the foods and with steaming the loss is minimal. (For example when broccoli is steamed, it retains 81% of its vitamin C. When it is cooked in water, it retains approximately 30%. When steamed, broccoli retains almost 89% of its flavonoids as opposed to when cooked in water it retains only 44% and when microwaved it retains only 3 %.) Several other factors make steaming appealing to include the retention of color, juices and freshness.

Unfortunately, there are some things that make steaming unappealing as a cooking choice, like the amount of time it takes compared to other ways of cooking and the fact that it has to be monitored, so that your water can be replenished when it evaporates. As well, there is typically no gravy left as can be by baking or frying.

Information that changes or influences your thoughts is just that – information; it's nothing personal

BOILING

Essentially, boiling sterilizes food, which is a great way to guarantee that we are not ingesting parasites, organisms and harmful substances from harvested food.

Normally, boiling doesn't change the flavor much in our foods and if you're like me and love green leafy vegetables like, mustard greens, run-ups, turnip greens, collards, cabbage, kale, spinach, chards, ramps and even broccoli (cauliflower too), boiling is a great way to soften these foods while adding flavor and making a really healthy meal with consumable juices when it's done.

When meat is boiled the fats and other indigestible components that are a part of meat usually dissipate into the water and can be drained off. Amongst the various important benefits of boiled food, we cannot ignore the digestibility factor. Boiling renders food items such as poultry and meat more digestible.

The fats, contained in the food items get easily dissolved in the boiling water, thus making the food healthy and easier to digest. Plus you've got a gravy left if you want it which is probably full of the nutrients that might have been boiled out of the meat or vegetables.

Besides the above mentioned traditional benefits of boiled foods, it must be noted that boiled food can be prepared in bulk and therefore, this method of cooking is ideal for large scale cooking and storage.

MICROWAVE

The quickest and probably most used method of food preparation is the grand ole microwave. And I'll go ahead and admit that I use it often and it is incredibly convenient at the end of a long day of work. The challenge for microwaved food however is fairly grand. The biggest negative of preparing food using a microwave is that it breaks the nutrients down from their natural state when exposed to the extreme and concentrated heat of the microwave for too long.

At the same time because most microwave cooking is short in terms of time, very often food has less exposure to sustained heat. For example, vitamins are preserved better in microwaving versus boiling or frying when the exposure is less than that of the other cooking methods When vegetables are cooked in boiling water some of the nutrients leech in to the water itself and if gravy is not to be made of the water then most likely it is drained off and the nutrients lost.

According to a Harvard University Health Study article from January 2015, "The cooking method that best retains nutrients is one that cooks *quickly, heats food for the shortest amount of time,* and uses *as little liquid as possible.* Microwaving meets those criteria."

"The first wealth is health."[16]

~Ralph Waldo Emerson

GRILLING

Although many of us think about grilling as a summer activity, there are those of us who love it so much that we've moved to particular locations across the country so we can grill year-round. There are so many benefits to grilling that it's not just about food anymore, but it has morphed into a world-wide-culture of social gatherings (especially at sporting events). Some of the other advantages to grilling occur when properly grilled meats burn a good deal of fat off of them when kissed directly by the grill flames. As well, there is a distinct flavor enhancement when food is grilled.

Most grills are efficient in terms of venting, which allows for moisture and air to circulate well inside the grill. Because of the ventilation, most modern grills versus open fire grilling, helps to retain taste. This air control also helps to keep the nutrients in meat and vegetables intact, which is vital to creating healthy meals.

Grilling is also cost efficient as cooking indoors can raise the indoor temperature in the kitchen by as much as 5-6 degrees (that impacts the comfort and thermostat indoors and your energy bill) and, depending on how much and what you are cooking, it can be much faster once the grill is on to get your food cooked and perhaps more of it.

The two downsides of grilling are first, it is not eco-friendly since you're burning a consumable (like wood chips, charcoal, wood or even gas) which can pose environmental concerns over the long haul. Secondly, if you are like some people who love their grilled and cooked foods done well (and some even like it dry and crispy) the risk of hydro-carbons ingestion is fairly high. Hydro-carbons have been shown to raise the risks for colorectal and stomach cancers.

SMOKED PRODUCTS

The major benefits of smoking food are that it kills bacteria and slows the growth of certain types of other bacteria. Smoking simply is a cooking style where a medium heat is used and often specific types of wood is used to infiltrate the fibers of the food to flavor it, cook it and preserve it. Smoking is an ancient form of food preparation that has been used for centuries and is even more popular today because of modern technology. Smoking used to be done in a concrete structure where meats in particularly were hung and left until the fire went out. Now we have gas/ propane powered smokers, a plethora of grills designed to smoke and even indoor electric smokers. Other benefits of smoking include the fact that it adds some flavor to most foods. It keeps the fat found in most meats from developing an unsavory taste which can happen in baking, broiling, and boiling.

Most often smoking adds a pleasing coloration to the food being smoked, and ultimately not so important in current society, but it helps preserves the meats and foods' storage life. The only prevalent negative is that *industrialized smoking of foods* has shown some carcinogenic traces in the intestinal tract of people who consumed high doses of foods smoked through the factory-manufactured smoked process. The key is smoking your food properly to avoid the negatives of this cooking style.

About eighty percent of the food on shelves of supermarkets today didn't exist 100 years ago."[17]

~ Larry McCleary

PALEO

Paleo eating is rather simple. The way it is most often described is eating anything a caveman could have gotten his or her hands on. Typically the foods are single ingredient foods which can be prepared in traditional ways but start out as a clean foods, (see Clean Eating)

"By cleansing your body on a regular basis and eliminating as many toxins as possible from your environment, your body can begin to heal itself, prevent disease, and become stronger and more resilient than you ever dreamed possible!"[18]

~ Dr. Edward Group III

VEGAN (PURE VEGETARIAN)

A pure vegetarian eating style is just that. With this eating style a person eats only nuts, legumes, grains, vegetable and fruit based foods. No meats, no dairy, no fish, insects and bugs, dairy based drinks are eaten or consumed – It is as plain as that.

PESCATARIAN

The Pescatarian only eats fish as means of protein from meats. No other meats are eaten. In addition they eat all of the fruits, vegetables, grains, legumes, eggs, and dairy that vegetarians typically consume.

VEGETARIAN

The vegetarian eats similarly to a vegan based eating plan already mentioned. The reason it is mentioned here is that there is a variation called a lactovegetarian who eats all that a vegetarian eats and adds cheese and dairy products to include eggs.

REGARDLESS OF HOW YOU CHOOSE TO EAT CONSIDER THIS:

Here are the things to skip while on whatever plan you choose for at least thirty days during your weight reduction efforts

- No wheat (except 1/2 cup brown rice)
- No artificial sweeteners (this includes all diet soda)
- No white sugar
- No alcohol
- No caffeine (only green tea)
- No dairy (except Greek yogurt)
- No meals between 8 p.m. to 8 a.m.

Chapter Fourteen

Managing Your Skin

While Reducing Your Weight

There is an issue related to weight loss that can be serious for those it affects and a potential deterrent for some if they are inclined to be well read on the subject of "weight loss." This is the issue of skin. When it comes to reducing one's weight, depending on how much weight and how fast the weight is reduced, skin may readjust and be stubborn to reduce in certain places. It can simply be so abundant that it creates a complete second layer of overlapping skin typically about the waist.

It is important to note that there is a difference between what often times is described as loose skin or fat that exists just below the surface of the skin and what is truly extra skin.

One quick way to gauge whether you are dealing with extra skin or whether you are dealing with loose skin is to actually grab some skin around your waist particularly, or to the right or left of your navel (bellybutton), and determine whether it is more than a half-inch thick. If that is the case then you are probably dealing with skin that is loose, rather than extra skin. So what is loose skin? Loose skin is typically skin that has adipose or fat cells underneath the actual skin. Of course fat, being an oily based substance, might just be the reason why the skin feels loose. When the skin is grabbed it is sliding over the adipose or fat cells right underneath the layer of skin. Another quick, distinguishing point between extra skin and loose skin is that loose skin tends to move a lot when you are active. Perhaps one might say it shakes, shutters, or wobbles.

Ultimately, when you get to this point in your weight management efforts, the fact that your skin feels this way might suggest that you are achieving your goals. As you continue to reduce the amount of fat in your body, there's a good chance that this type of loose skin hiding adipose tissue/fat will go away and the skin will return to a normal elasticity and not become extra skin.

The idea here is that surgical procedures could in fact remove the extra skin, however, at all costs, managing the weight reduction process is probably key to avoiding the measure of surgery related to skin removal. Towards the end of this section some ideas from various information repositories will be shared for you to consider as you look to manage the potential concerns with loose and extra skin.

Please know that I am not anti-surgery and if it is warranted, and you are comfortable with it, and you can afford it, then I fully advocate its occurrence. On the other hand, there will be permanent reminders of the extra skin's removal that may cause more psychological concern than the skin itself. Additionally, I have had to deal with loose skin and what has worked for me may not work for you. However, as you consider the data be weary of giving up before you have exhausted all means.

To gauge whether you are dealing with extra skin perform the same test, previously mentioned. If you find that your skin is very thin, similar to what you might find in between your knuckles joints on the backside of your hand, or on the underside of your wrist, palm side, and it is more than a handful then you may be dealing with extra skin.

So, let us talk first about how to manage your prevention efforts when it comes to extra skin as you engage in your efforts to reduce your weight. In an effort to keep skin taunt, that is to say tight in a manner that tends to loosely fit your body as you reduce your weight, there must be toned muscle in the places where you reduce your adipose tissue. What am I saying?

As you reduce the fat cells in your body, you must be working on developing muscle tone, so that when the fat is "burned off," your skin gets its form or shape from the muscle structure beneath it. This is true of your abdomen, your chest/breast, arms, buttock, calves, upper-outer part of your back and your inner thighs.

This ideally occurs when you are not rapidly reducing your weight – so that your muscular structure can keep up with the reduction. If you reduce your weight incredibly fast without the proper regiment of fiber development in your muscles – then there is a good chance that you will in fact end up with extra/excess skin.

So, can you maintain a controlled process for targeting fat and not having it happen so rapidly so as to create excess skin? Well, the answer is yes based on some specific studies conducted with random participants. The idea of controlling weight reduction is not only possible but may be key in managing your skin concerns.

In short, whenever you can control the rate in which you reduce your weight, it is helpful in that you can keep your body from rapid weight reduction which usually and most often leads to the excess skin.

So what can you do? (The following information and ideas come from varying sources that include: verywell.com, webmd.com, womenshealthmag.com, prevention.com and everydayhealth.com, as well as The Boston Medical Center, and The Cleveland Clinic.)

1. NUMBER ONE is the number one method on the list. The best way to reduce excess skin ahead of its development is to workout using weights. That's right, building toned muscle under your skin will help keep it taunt while you reduce the fat throughout your body. Over time, given the appropriate vitamins and nutrients. Your Skin can retain its elasticity and will shrink in ratio to the reduced weight. As long as it reduction is slow and controlled, it will maintain its healthy elasticity.
2. Any manipulation of skin and or muscle stimulates blood circulation. Ultimately, if the skin has good blood flow there is a good chance that the skin will be healthier. Salt scrubs, or other kinds of scrubs that specifically target skin that could become loose, excessive, or flabby might enhance the skins blood flow and thus its elasticity. At a minimum, salt scrubs seem to work best if done at least 4 to 5 times weekly. While showering and or even up to two times a day is good. (According to some sources mineral scrubs can create enhanced results; this includes scrubs that contain sand.)
3. If you are reducing your weight by a significant amount, one of the things you may want to consider so you can avoid having cosmetic procedures is to use skin firming lotions to tighten skin. These lotions typically provide nutrients designed to increase the collagen as well as the elastin throughout your skin tend to be beneficial. Without advocating specific products, or nutrients, suffice it to say that products with aloe-vera, vitamin K, and vitamin E, are going to be the best options as they are all related to collagen and elastin development.
4. Another great technique for managing loose, excessive, or potentially flabby skin is to prevent it. Part of the prevention process is to be properly hydrated. Hydration simply involves the infusion of water. Of course, the human body. Depending on which study you observe is 60 to 72% comprised of water. At these percentages, the body tends to function at its optimal

levels. So, being sure to add water to your daily regimen can be nothing but healthy for your skin.

5. Avoid extensive tanning and remaining in the sun (i.e., at the beach every day, vs. one week or three or four days with a break in between). This also goes for being in the pool every day, for more than two hours at a time. The sun as well as chlorinated water has a tendency to loosen the skin breaking down its elasticity and creating things like crow's feet, wrinkles around the mouth, and excessive lines in the shrinking stomach, etc. This limitation also applies to tanning booths as well as outdoor sunlight.
6. Avoid using extremely hot water in showering. How can you tell when your water is too hot? Ask yourself, "Do I like hot showers?" If the answer is yes, then taper back the water until it is warm, instead of hot. The concern is that the hotter the water, the higher the risk of stripping the skin of its natural oils. Your natural oils help retain your skin's moisture and contribute to its healthiness and elasticity.
7. Oil that is extracted from almonds has been suggested in the literature to be an alternative for tightening and conditioning the skin from a loose and stretched condition. A half a teaspoon rubbed across the abdomen nightly, (hips too) creates very soft skin and helps with making the skin taunt.
8. In the same way that you would use an astringent for your face; the option to use an astringent, particularly on your stomach can have the same effect. When using an astringent it typically tightens the skin. According to some home remedy sources of creative and perhaps inexpensive astringent includes honey, rosemary and witch hazel.
9. Very often for those concerned with their skin, a cosmetic mask can be used to tighten and make their skin taut. In an effort to be or remain logical it might make sense that using a mask on, particularly the stomach area could tighten the skin there. I have no evidence for this; (that is, using an egg white mask, as you would for facial, on your stomach. Then

rinsing it off as you would with the facial mask,) however, I am including it because I have seen it in at least three different sources. You will have to evaluate for yourself.

10. In the effort to manage food and its impact on your skin, you will have to consider what is in your food. Of course you want to manage your food intake anyway. It becomes even more important to manage the ingredients of your food when concerned about your skin. Managing your ingredients means that you manage fat, manage chemicals, manage the pathogens in your food, and even the cleanliness of your food.

    Of course that means dirt on your naturally grown foods, but more than that, eating cleanly, which is eating single ingredient foods to include raw vegetables and fruits. (Ask anyone whose skin reacts to the sugar they intake, and they will tell you that what you put in your body definitely affects your skin.) Eating raw, single ingredient foods like vegetables and fruit helps you avoid foods that might have the proteins and other good nutrients denatured out of them by cooking.

11. An otherwise poisonous extract of castor beans, is a beneficial oil when it used externally. It along with lemon juice provides a nutritional supplement to your skin. The way in which it's supposed to work is that when used nightly for most people, it tightens skin perfectly on the abdomen and around the hips and under the arms. One source even recommends mixing a tad bit of lavender oil with the castor oil and lemon juice to obtain the same results of tightening the skin in the abdomen except the lavender adds a relaxing aroma.

Ultimately, managing, preventing and dealing with potentially excessive skin, loose skin, and stretch marks can be a seemingly daunting task. Not being a dermatologist, the ideas I presented are suggestive in nature with the idea that some of them may take longer than you are willing to wait. Several of them in the literature suggest that it takes months to see the results. However, in light of the unconventional, it would seem that trying any one of these potential solutions might be less expensive, less painful, and certainly less scarring than the alternative.

EPILOGUE

I had finished this manuscript some four months earlier and held on to it. It was as if I was waiting for something. When it happened, the flood of emotions, sadness and regret was unstoppable. I wasn't sad because of the death, nor was I sad as a result of the loss. I was sad that my dear friend chose to do nothing about his hypertension, knowing full well the consequences. I was sad for his kids who were left without their champion and greatest advocate. I was sad that his encouraging spouse was left without her best friend in light of her ongoing encouragement for him to take better care of himself. Never making it to that fourth decade and watching those last moments of consciousness slip away weighed heavily on my mind over the next few days and then I realized what was missing in this book, The SENSE OF URGENCY. It was as if I had missed a crucial point that was to help you gain your catalyst to do what you've read,

Now!

Your moments are but few in life; on average you have 21,000 days' worth of them. That's if you're fortunate; and then moments later I was searching for something unrelated and a series of clicks led me to the following blog. I read it and discovered the impact of my thoughts conveyed directly and precisely. With respect to those who practice existentialism, it is not my philosophy, and if that is what you choose, I hope it works for you long-term. On the other hand if in the next few moments, what you read is a basis of what is shared in that community, then I welcome it into my thought process and embrace the active part of seeking to live fully in light of the inevitable truth of death that this truth/philosophy espouses.

It is my desire that as you read it, you will be more inspired than you already are to take charge of your life, perhaps you will join us for one of our annual seminars to actively change, secure and live out your purpose, dreams and your destiny as a fulfilled healthy human being.

"Hour of the mayfly": adapted from Tim Rayner, Philosophy for Change

September 2, 2013

Ever stared death in the eye? If you've not had the pleasure, like Pfc. Don Doll here in this short story, I recommend a thought experiment. Imagine that, right now, you are teletransported to the heart of a military conflict. Ker-bang. One moment you are surfing the internet, next moment you are knee deep in the mud with bullets hissing through the elephant grass about you. An explosion throws you down. S#:+ just got real. You could be dead in an instant.

You want to run, cry, and call for your mother. But there is no escape. You crouch low in the grass, taking deep breaths. Your heart is booming in your chest. You are alive – for the moment. This simple truth has enveloped your entire consciousness. How strange it is that you didn't reflect on this before, you think. Why, all your life, you've been stumbling about as if in a dream. Now, all you can think is: I'm still here! Life is not an abstract concept. You are living it, right now.

Death is in the moment too. Amid the explosions, shots and screams, the truth of human mortality is

> shockingly clear. Death is not something that lies far off in the distance, like the closing scene of a movie or the final chapter of a book. Death can come anytime, anyplace. The bullets are in flight, the bombs are descending. The hand of death may be on you now.
>
> This is the truth of human mortality. Face this truth and it will change you.
>
> What is true on the battlefield is true for us all. No one knows when their time is coming. You can exercise, eat nutritious foods and steer clear of stressful environments. It may lessen your chances of cancer and disease in the long term, but it won't change a thing when a learner driver misses a red light or a once-in-a-lifetime earthquake brings the roof down on your head.

Granted, earthquakes are rare and the chances of a fatal accident are slim if you take appropriate precautions. But this doesn't change the fact that you do not control the time of your death. Death may come in sixty years or sixty seconds from now. The reality is, none of us know. This is what it means to confront personal mortality.

Confronting death is like a shock of cold water to the face. The presence of death shatters our fascination with superficial things in life. Suddenly we are wide awake at existence ground zero. We start asking questions. We start thinking seriously about who we are and how we are living. And we start asking what we are really capable of achieving in the time that we have left to us.

The philosophers Friedrich Nietzsche, Martin Heidegger, Jean-Paul Sartre, and Albert Camus were so impressed with the transformative power of death that they made confronting death central to their philosophical way of living. Death, they argued, brings life and its possibilities into focus. In the process, it reveals what we are ultimately capable of being. Heidegger argues that confronting death brings to light 'the totality of our potentiality-for-Being'. In a moment of vision, we grasp our full sphere of potential – a realm of potential that is ours and ours alone, that we may or may not take advantage of. We catch a glimpse of our whole person, our total capacity to exist. And we experience an obligation to live up to our capacity before death takes it away.

Mostly we shirk the obligation. It is too hard to bear. We retreat into comfort zones. We shy away from what we are capable of being. The novel that you have stowed half-finished in the bottom drawer of your desk. The broken relationship that you could heal with a few gentle words, words that you've never found a way of saying. The mountains of the Himalayas – haven't they been calling you for years? We all live with a sense of potential sealed beneath the ice of everyday life – dreams and desires that we want to claim, but that we feel incapable of making our own.

> *Take an axe and break the ice. Confronting death can be a frightening experience. But it focuses you on your unique possibilities and liberates your passion for change*
>
> *CLE*

Often when people stand up and take hold of life, they look back on their previous state and ask: 'What was I afraid of?' A human life is longer than most. Compare it to the life of the mayfly, the tiny cousin to the dragonfly. The mayfly lays its eggs near lakes and streams in North America. It spends the day buzzing merrily about sunny banks and cool waters, mating and feeding on algae all day, if it's lucky, for this is all a mayfly gets – one day or less. A mayfly can die within thirty minutes of bursting from its aquatic naiad stage into an adult form. To watch the mayfly spawn and die is a potent reminder of the transience of life and our necessary human finitude.

Imagine being born a mayfly. Or, imagine being born a mayfly with the knowledge and intelligence that you have today, knowing that life is drastically limited and death is literally imminent. Would you flutter to the ground and lie there twitching in despair, waiting for a passing predator to snap you up? Or would you take stock of the numerous possibilities for pleasure and experience that are granted a mayfly in the course of its short life and say: 'Yes! There has never been a better time for living!'

It would be foolish to do otherwise. The key to taking something marvelous from the shortest span of existence is to affirm what you have and live.

To enjoy the rewards of a pure-existing life, we need to face death at each opportunity. When you wake up tomorrow, take a moment to reflect on how great it is that you have lived to see another day. Say: 'thank you'. Life is better when it is lived in the presence of death. Over breakfast, ask yourself: 'Would I choose Wheaties for my final meal? Is this coffee the best of all espressos? Would I even drink it if I only had an hour to live?' Keep mortality in mind as you commute to the office. Who knows, by the time you get to work, you may have decided that you are ready for change.

Affirm life in its contingency and finitude. Affirm each moment as a critical juncture – a moment ripe for decision, for determining the way that you live. Live life as a flash of light in the void. Rejoice in the gift of existence and revel in its profound possibilities. Live Fully and Healthily!

BEGIN YOUR JOURNEY NOW!

www.youwillseeresults.com

Appendix

SURVEY: Used for Data Collection:

A Simple Survey: Can be Traded for One Coaching Session

1. How would you describe your pre "weight loss life" – (i.e. Discipline, willingness, awareness of healthiness, eating habits, etc?)

2. How would you describe your life now related to understanding healthiness?

3. Where were you when you made the choice to change?

4. Describe the moment when you made the decision, what triggered it?

5. How did you get started?

6. What made you stick with it?

7. Did you influence anyone else to join you?

8. How do you feel now?

9. How long has it been since you changed your lifestyle?

10. Was there weekly changes or did it happen without fan-fare and you suddenly you noticed?

11. What do you do now that you either couldn’t then or didn’t want to do then?

12. What do think would have happened if you had simply tried to" lose weight" rather than get rid of fat and be healthier?

13. What do you think would have happened if you did nothing?

Comments:

Peer-Reviewed Research References

1. Dubuc GR, Havel PJ et al. Changes of serum leptin and endocrine and metabolic parameters after 7 days of energy restriction in men and women. Metabolism. 1998 Apr;47(4):429-34.
2. Ngondi JL, Etoundi BC, Nyangono CB, Mbofung CM, Oben JE, "IGOB131, a novel seed extract of the West African plant Irvingia gabonensis, significantly reduces body weight and improves metabolic parameters in overweight humans in a randomized double-blind placebo controlled investigation," Lipids Health Dis. 2009 Mar 2;8:7
3. Dirlewanger M, et al. Effects of short-term carbohydrate or fat overfeeding on energy expenditure and plasma leptin concentrations in healthy female subjects. Int J Obes Relat Metab Disord. 2000 Nov;24(11):1413-8.
4. Ahima RS, Flier JS. Leptin. Annu Rev Physiol. 2000;62:413-37. Review.
5. Bowles L, Kopelman P. Leptin: of mice and men? J. Clin Pathol 2001 Jan;54(1):1-3
6. Ahima RS, et al. Leptin regulation of neuroendocrine systems. Front Neuroendocrinology 2000 Jul;21(3):263-307.
7. Van Dijk G. The role of leptin in regulation of energy balance and adiposity. J. Neuroendocrinol 2001 Oct;13(10):913-21.
8. Rosenbaum M et. al. Low dose leptin administration reverses effects of sustained weight-reduction on energy expenditure

and circulating concentrations of thyroid hormones. J. Clin Endocrinol Metab (2002) 87:2391-2394.

9. Eamon P. RAFFERTY 1, Alastair R. WYLIE, Chris T. ELLIOTT, Olivier P. CHEVALLIER, David J. GRIEVE, Brian D. GREEN. In Vitro and In Vivo Effects of Natural Putative Secretagogues of Glucagon-Like Peptide-1 (GLP-1). Sci Pharm. 2011; 79: 615–621
10. Kennedy A et al. The metabolic significance of leptin in humans: gender-based differences in relationship to adiposity, insulin sensitivity, and energy expenditure. J. Clin Endocrinol Metab. 1997 Apr;82(4):1293-300.
11. Havel PJ et al. Relationship of plasma leptin to plasma insulin and adiposity in normal weight and overweight women: effects of dietary fat content and sustained weight loss. J. Clin Endocrinol Metab. 1996 Dec;81(12):4406-13.
12. Doucet E et al. Changes in energy expenditure and substrate oxidation resulting from weight loss in obese men and women: is there an important contribution of leptin? J Clin Endocrinol Metab. 2000 Apr;85(4):1550-6.
13. Nicklas BJ et al. Gender differences in the response of plasma leptin concentrations to weight loss in obese older individuals. Obes Res. 1997 Jan;5(1):62-8.
14. Racette SB, Kohrt WM et al. Response of serum leptin concentrations to 7 d of energy restriction in centrally obese African Americans with impaired or diabetic glucose tolerance. Am J Clin Nutr. 1997 Jul;66(1):33-7.
15. Havel PJ et al. High-fat meals reduce 24-h circulating leptin concentrations in women. Diabetes. 1999 Feb;48(2):334-41.
16. Boden G et al. Effect of fasting on serum leptin in normal human subjects. J Clin Endocrinol Metab. 1996 Sep;81(9):3419-23.
17. Miyawaki T et al. Clinical implications of leptin and its potential humoral regulators in long-term low-calorie diet therapy for obese humans. Eur J Clin Nutr. 2002 Jul;56(7):593600.
18. Carantoni M et al. Can changes in plasma insulin concentration explain the variability in leptin response to weight loss in obese

women with normal glucose tolerance? J Clin Endocrinol Metab. 1999 Mar;84(3):869-72.

19. Zimmet P. Serum leptin concentration, obesity, and insulin resistance in Western Samoans: cross sectional study. BMJ. 1996 Oct 19;313(7063):965-9.
20. Tuominen et al. Leptin and thermogenesis in humans. Acta Physiol Scand. 1997 May;160(1):83-7.
21. Keim NL, Stern JS, Havel PJ. Relation between circulating leptin concentrations and appetite during a prolonged, moderate energy deficit in women. Am J Clin Nutr. 1998 Oct;68(4):794-801.
22. Haluzik M et al. The influence of short-term fasting on serum leptin levels, and selected hormonal and metabolic parameters in morbidly obese and lean females. Endocr Res. 2001 FebMay;27(1-2):251-60.
23. Mars M et al. Leptin and insulin responses to a four-day energy-deficient diet in men with different weight history. Int J Obes Relat Metab Disord. 2003 May;27(5):574-81.
24. Pratley RE et al. Plasma leptin responses to fasting in Pima Indians. Am J Physiol. 1997 Sep;273(3 Pt 1):E644-9.
25. Okazaki T et al. Effects of mild aerobic exercise and a mild hypocaloric diet on plasma leptin in sedentary women. Clin Exp Pharmacol Physiol. 1999 May-Jun;26(5-6):415-20.
26. Mars M et al. Fasting leptin and appetite responses induced by a 4-day 65%-energy-restricted diet. Int J Obes (Lond). 2006 Jan;30(1):122-8.
27. Kolaczynski JW. Responses of leptin to short-term fasting and refeeding in humans: a link with ketogenesis but not ketones themselves. Diabetes. 1996 Nov;45(11):1511-5.
28. Kolaczynski JW. Response of leptin to short-term and prolonged overfeeding in humans. J Clin Endocrinol Metab. 1996 Nov;81(11):4162-5.
29. Palesty JA. The goldilocks paradigm of starvation and refeeding. Nutr Clin Pract. 2006 Apr;21(2):147-54. Review.
30. Turek VF, Trevaskis JL, Levin BE, Dunn-Meynell AA, Irani B, Gu G, Wittmer C, Griffin PS, Vu C, Parkes DG, Roth JD.

Mechanisms of amylin/leptin synergy in rodent models. Amylin Pharmaceuticals, Inc., 9360 Towne Centre Drive, San Diego, California 92121, USA.

31. Reseland JE et al. Effect of long-term changes in diet and exercise on plasma leptin concentrations. Am J Clin Nutr. 2001 Feb;73(2):240-5.
32. Romon M et al. Leptin response to carbohydrate or fat meal and association with subsequent satiety and energy intake. Am J Physiol. 1999 Nov;277(5 Pt 1):E855-61.
33. Van Aggel-Leijssen DP et al. Regulation of average 24h human plasma leptin level; the influence of exercise and physiological changes in energy balance. Int J Obes Relat Metab Disord. 1999 Feb;23(2):151-8.
34. Hamann A, Matthaei S. Regulation of energy balance by leptin. Exp Clin Endocrinol Diabetes. 1996;104(4):293-300. Review.
35. Ahima RS et al. Role of leptin in the neuroendocrine response to fasting. Nature. 1996 Jul 18;382(6588):250-2.
36. Meinders AE et al. Leptin. Neth J Med. 1996 Dec;49(6):247-52. Review.
37. Girard J. Is leptin the link between obesity and insulin resistance? Diabetes Metab. 1997 Sep;23 Suppl 3:16-24. Review.
38. Nedvidkova J. Leptin. Cesk Fysiol. 1997 Dec;46(4):182-8. Review.
39. Spitzweg C, Joba W, Heufelder AE. Leptin – new knowledge on the pathogenesis of obesity. Med Klin (Munich). 1998 Aug 15;93(8):478-85. Review.
40. Clark CD, Bassett B, Burge MR. Effects of kelp supplementation on thyroid function in euthyroid subjects. Endocr Pract. 2003 Sep-Oct;9(5):363-9.
41. Maffei M, Halaas J et al. Leptin levels in human and rodent: measurement of plasma leptin and ob RNA in obese and weight-reduced subjects. Nat Med. 1995 Nov;1(11):1155-61.
42. Ferruccio Santini, et al. Acute exogenous TSH administration stimulates leptin secretion in vivo. Eur J Endocrinol July 1, 2010 163 63-67.

43. Wolf G. Leptin: the weight-reducing plasma protein encoded by the obese gene. Nutr Rev. 1996 Mar;54(3):91-3. Review.
44. Boden G et al. Effect of fasting on serum leptin in normal human subjects. J Clin Endocrinol Metab. 1996 Sep;81(9):3419-23.
45. Levin BE, Routh VH. Role of the brain in energy balance and obesity. Am J Physiol. 1996 Sep;271(3 Pt 2):R491-500. Review.
46. Kim JH, Kang SA, Han SM, Shim I. Comparison of the antiobesity effects of the protopanaxadiol – and protopanaxatriol-type saponins of red ginseng. Phytother Res. 2009 Jan;23(1):78-85.
47. Yang CY, et al. Anti-diabetic effects of Panax notoginseng saponins and its major anti-hyperglycemic components. J Ethnopharmacol. 2010 Jul 20;130(2):231-6. Epub 2010 May 8.
48. Smith SR. The endocrinology of obesity. Endocrinol Metab Clin North Am. 1996 Dec;25(4):921-42. Review.
49. Hwa JJ et al. Intracerebroventricular injection of leptin increases thermogenesis and mobilizes fat metabolism in ob/ob mice. Horm Metab Res. 1996 Dec;28(12):659-63.
50. Wing RR et al. Relationship between weight loss maintenance and changes in serum leptin levels. Horm Metab Res. 1996 Dec;28(12):698-703.
51. Martinez JA, Fruhbek G. Regulation of energy balance and adiposity: a model with new approaches. Rev Esp Fisiol. 1996 Dec;52(4):255-8. Review.
52. Schwartz MW, Seeley RJ. The new biology of body weight regulation. J Am Diet Assoc. 1997 Jan;97(1):54-8; quiz 59-60. Review.
53. Rohner-Jeanrenaud E, Jeanrenaud B. Central nervous system and body weight regulation. Ann Endocrinol (Paris). 1997;58(2):137-42. Review.
54. Blum WF. Leptin: the voice of the adipose tissue. Horm Res. 1997;48 Suppl 4:2-8. Review.
55. Weigle DS et al. Effect of fasting, refeeding, and dietary fat restriction on plasma leptin levels. J Clin Endocrinol Metab. 1997 Feb;82(2):561-5.

56. Jenkins AB et al. Carbohydrate intake and short-term regulation of leptin in humans. Diabetologia. 1997 Mar;40(3):348-51.
57. Westerterp-Plantenga MS. Green tea catechins, caffeine and body-weight regulation. Physiol Behav. 2010 Apr 26;100(1):42-6. Epub 2010 Feb 13.
58. Malmstrom R et al. Insulin increases plasma leptin concentrations in normal subjects and patients with NIDDM. Diabetologia. 1996 Aug;39(8):993-6.
59. Wisse BE et al. Effect of prolonged moderate and severe energy restriction and refeeding on plasma leptin concentrations in obese women. Am J Clin Nutr. 1999 Sep;70(3):321-30.
60. Fogteloo AJ et al. Effects of recombinant human leptin treatment as an adjunct of moderate energy restriction on body weight, resting energy expenditure and energy intake in obese humans. Diabetes Nutr Metab. 2003 Apr;16(2):109-14.
61. Coleman RA et al. Nutritional regulation of leptin in humans. Diabetologia. 1999 42(6): 639-46
62. Evans et al. Carbohydrate and fat have different effects on plasma leptin concentrations and adipose tissue leptin production. Clin Sci (Lond). 2001 May;100(5):493-8.
63. Schwartz MW et al. Model for the regulation of energy balance and adiposity by the central nervous system. Am J Clin Nutr. 1999. 69: 584-596
64. Jequier E and L Tappy. Regulation of body weight in humans. Physiol Rev. 1999. 79: 451-480
65. Levine AS and CK Billington. Do circulating leptin concentrations reflect body adiposity or energy flux? Am J Cline Nutr. 1998. 68: 761-762
66. Jequier E. Leptin signaling, adiposity, and energy balance. Ann N Y Acad Sci. 2002. Jun;967:379-88. Review.
67. Havel, PJ. Mechanisms Regulating Leptin Production: Implications for Control of Energy Balance. American Journal of Clinical Nutrition, (Editorial) 70: 305-306, 1999.
68. Havel, PJ. Peripheral signals conveying metabolic information to the brain: short-term and long-term regulation of food in-take

and energy homeostasis. Exp Biol Med (Maywood) 2001;226: 963-977.

69. Havel, Peter J. Role of Adipose Tissue in Body Weight Regulation: Mechanisms Regulating Leptin Production and Energy Balance. Proceedings of the Nutrition Society 59: 359-371, 2000.
70. Heymsfield et al. Recombinant leptin for weight loss in obese and lean adults: a randomized, controlled, dose-escalation trial. JAMA. 1999 Oct 27;282(16):1568-75.
71. Welt C, et al. Recombinant human leptin in women with hypothalamic amenorrhea. N. Engl. J. Med. 2004;351:987 – 997.
72. Reseland JE et al. Effect of long-term changes in diet and exercise on plasma leptin concentrations. Am J Clin Nutr. 2001 Feb;73(2):240-5.
73. Chu NF et al. Dietary and lifestyle factors in relation to plasma leptin concentrations among normal weight and overweight men. Int J Obes Relat Metab Disord. 2001 Jan;25(1):106-14.
74. Koutsari C et al. Plasma leptin is influenced by diet composition and exercise. Int J Obes Relat Metab Disord. 2003 Aug;27(8):901-6.
75. Hussein GM, et al. Mate tea (Ilex paraguariensis) promotes satiety and body weight lowering in mice: involvement of glucagon-like peptide-1. Biol Pharm Bull. 2011;34(12):1849-55.
76. Dyck DJ. Leptin sensitivity in skeletal muscle is modulated by diet and exercise. Exerc Sport Sci Rev. 2005 Oct;33(4):18994. Review.
77. Rosenbaum et al. Low-dose leptin reverses skeletal muscle, autonomic, and neuroendocrine adaptations to maintenance of reduced weight. J Clin Invest. 2005 Dec;115(12):3579-86
78. Dor AF, Langwith C, Tan E. A heavy burden: The individual costs of being overweight and obese in the United States. The George Washington University School of Public Health and Health Services Department of Health Policy, 2010.
79. The National Institute of Diabetes and Digestive and Kidney Diseases (NIDDK) conducts and supports a broad range of basic and clinical obesity research. More information about obesity research is available at http://www.obesityresearch. nih.gov.

80. Hour of the mayfly" : adapted from Tim Rayner, Philosophy for Change, September 2, 2013 By http://philosophyforchange.wordpress.com/author/timrayner/

OBESITY and METABOLIC SYNDROME

1. How are overweight and obesity diagnosed? National Heart, Lung, and Blood Institute website. *http://www.nhlbi.nih.gov/health/health-topics/topics/obe/ diagnosis.html.* Updated July 13, 2012. Accessed October 4, 2012.
2. How is metabolic syndrome diagnosed? National Heart, Lung, and Blood Institute website. *http://www.nhlbi.nih.gov/ health/health-topics/topics/ms/diagnosis.html.* Updated November 3, 2011. Accessed October 4, 2012.
3. Ten leading causes of death and injury, 2009. Centers for Disease Control and Prevention. Web-based Injury Statistics Query and Reporting System (WISQARS). 2011. *http://www.cdc.gov/injury/wisqars/LeadingCauses.html.*
4. National diabetes statistics, 2011. National Diabetes Information Clearinghouse website. *http://diabetes.niddk.nih. gov/dm/pubs/statistics.* Updated December 6, 2011. Accessed July 26, 2012.
5. Diabetes overview. National Diabetes Information Clearinghouse website. *http://diabetes.niddk.nih.gov/dm/pubs/ overview.* Updated April 4, 2012. Accessed May 15, 2012.
6. Obesity and cancer risk. National Cancer Institute. *http://www.cancer.gov/cancertopics/factsheet/Risk/obesity.* Updated January 3, 2012. Accessed September 26, 2012.
7. Institute of Medicine and National Research Council. Weight Gain during Pregnancy: Reexamining the Guidelines. Washington, D.C.: The National Academies Press; 2009. *http://www.ncbi.nlm.nih.gov/books/*

ASPARTAME & ARTIFICIAL SWEETENERS

1. The Sugar Association. What is aspartame? *http://www.sugar.org/'/other-sweeteners/artificial-sweeteners/#aspartame* (Last accessed 2013-09-24)
2. European Patent Application EP0036258. Process for producing aspartame. *http://www.freepatentsonline.com/ EP0036258.html* (Last accessed 2013-09-24)
3. Qing Yang. Gain weight by "going diet?" Artificial sweeteners and the neurobiology of sugar cravings: Neuroscience 2010. The Yale Journal of Biology and Medicine. June 2010. *http://www.ncbi.nlm.nih.gov/pmc/articles/PMC2892765/*
4. Dorway. Formaldehyde: Not a Food Product. *http://dorway.com/aspartame-the-bad-news-repost/formaldehyde/* (Last accessed 2013-09-24)
5. Martin H. Fischer. The Toxic Effects of Formaldehyde and Formalin. The Journal of Experimental Medicine. February 1, 1905. doi: 10.1084/jem.6.4-6.487. *http://jem.rupress.org/content/6/4-6/487.abstract*
6. Dorway. Aspartame History. *http://dorway.com/history-ofaspartame/* (Last accessed 2013-09-24)

FOODS

1. *http://www.redbookmag.com/health-wellness/advice/snacks-forweight-loss_-22#comments 2013*
2. *http://www.redbookmag.com/health-wellness/advice/foods-thatreduce-bloating-9*

QUOTES

1. James Allen http://www.goodreads.com/quotes/502371-the-world-steps-aside-for-the-man-who-knows-where- James Allen, July 12, 2017 (adapted from a version attributed to Ralph Waldo

Emerson - "The world makes way for the man who knows where he is going."

2. Moliere`, https://www.brainyquote.com/quotes/quotes/m/moliere138703.html, Moliere` French Playwright, January 15, 1622 - February 17, 1673
3. Rollo May, https://cnx.org/contents/UQr0_DQ3@1/Viktor-Frankl-Rollo-May-and-Ex
4. Scriptures taken from the Holy Bible, New International Version®, NIV®. Copyright © 1973, 1978, 1984, 2011 by Biblica, Inc.™ Used by permission of Zondervan. All rights reserved worldwide. www.zondervan.com The "NIV" and "New International Version" are trademarks registered in the United States Patent and Trademark Office by Biblica, Inc.™
5. Victor Hugo, https://recoveringfed.com/tag/victor-hugo/ July 12, 2016
6. Andrew Jackson, http://www.beliefnet.com/quotes/inspiration/a/andrew-jackson/take-time-to-deliberate-but-when-the-time-for-act.aspx January, 3, 2017
7. Norman Augustine, https://essayforum.com/writing/motivation-almost-beat-mere-talent-61629/ January 14, 2015
8. Although many have attributed this quote to Mother Teresa, the website which is an extension of her work denies that she has said this - http://www.motherteresa.org/08_info/Quotesf.html#1a
9. 2007 Einstein: A Biography by Jürgen Neffe, Translator: Shelley Frisch (Translated from German to English), (Copyright 2005, Translation Copyright 2007), Chapter 19: From Barbaria to Dollaria; Einstein's America, Quote Page 369, Footnote 39: Quote Page 431, Published by Farrar, Straus, and Giroux, New York. (Verified on paper) (Original quote was not Albert Einstein but through translation was attributed to him)
10. William Purkey, quoteinvestigator.com/2014/02/02/dance/ July 19, 2016
11. Arthur Shoppenhauer is often given credit for the first interpretation of this quote in 1819. However it not exactly what he said and various others to include: Charles Lyell Louis

Agassiz J. Marion Sims and Apocryphal have been responsible for versions of it.
http://quoteinvestigator.com/2016/11/18/truth-stages/
July 19, 2017

12. Jim Rohn, http://www.goodreads.com/quotes/905713-take-care-of-your-body-it-s-the-only-place-you July 17, 2017
13. Nelson Mandela, http://aboutthree.com/blog/times-management-managements-time/ March 14, 2015
14. Vince Lombardi, https://medium.com/@steveagyei65/the-difference-between-a-successful-person-and-others-is-not-a-lack-of-strength-not-a-lack-of-2fe0a4a7fffd November 2, 2016
15. Katie Leah F., MD Conversation during her edits to the original manuscript May 13, 2017
16. Ralph Waldo Emerson http://www.huffingtonpost.com/susan-blumenthal/the-first-wealth-is-healt_b_141108.html July 12, 2017
17. Larry McCoy http://www.goodreads.com/quotes/353990-about-eighty-percent-of-the-food-on-shelves-of-supermarkets July 1 2013
18. Dr. Edward Group III http://healthy-ojas.com/systems/reflexology-benefits.html January 18, 2011

GENERAL RESEARCH

1. 2008 Physical Activity Guidelines for Americans
   http://www.health.gov/paguidelines
2. Action for Health in Diabetes (Look AHEAD) Trial
   https://www.lookaheadtrial.org
3. BMI Calculator
   http://www.nhlbi.nih.gov/guidelines/obesity/BMI/bmicalc.htm
4. Dietary Guidelines for Americans, 2010
   http://www.health.gov/DietaryGuidelines
5. MyPlate
   http://www.choosemyplate.gov
6. National Cancer Institute *http://www.cancer.gov*

7. National Diabetes Education Program
   http://www.yourdiabetesinfo.org
8. National Diabetes Information Clearinghouse
   http://www.diabetes.niddk.nih.gov
9. National Digestive Diseases Information Clearinghouse
   http://www.digestive.niddk.nih.gov
10. National Institute of Arthritis and Musculoskeletal and Skin Diseases
    http://www.niams.nih.gov
11. National Kidney Disease Education Program
    http://nkdep.nih.gov
12. U.S. Department of Agriculture Nutrition Website
    http://www.nutrition.gov

Eat less from a box and more from the earth

Take care of your body, it's the only place you have to live![12]

~Jim Rohn

www.ingramcontent.com/pod-product-compliance
Ingram Content Group UK Ltd.
Pitfield, Milton Keynes, MK11 3LW, UK
UKHW041946190726
13854UKWH00004B/1820